Changing Times:

A Nurse's Journey

Changing Times:

A Nurse's Journey

Pat Pickard

Illustrated by Pat McCarthy

© Pat Pickard

Published by Byron Press

ISBN 978-0-9569502-0-8

A CIP catalogue record for this book is available from the British Library.

Cover illustration by Pat McCarthy

Prepared and printed by:

York Publishing Services Ltd
64 Hallfield Road
Layerthorpe
York YO31 7ZQ

Tel: 01904 431213

Website: www.yps-publishing.co.uk

Dedication

For Steve who is always there for me,
and also the late Eileen Makinson –
a dear friend for over sixty years.

Acknowledgements

My thanks are due to former colleagues Joan Knight and Anne Nickson; to Maggie Awty-Jones for interpreting my notes; to Pat McCarthy whose illustrations brought my past to life, and finally to my husband Steve for his help and unfailing patience.

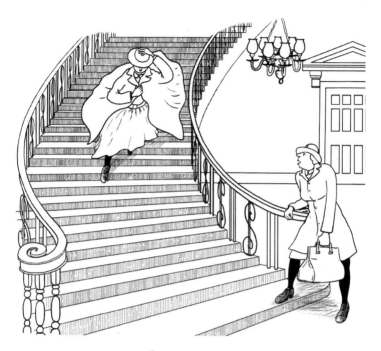

Chapter 1

It was raining as I walked up the long drive to the large imposing Victorian mansion. The air of January gloom was not dispelled by the overgrown rhododendrons dripping on my head. I pressed the bell and stood back looking at the stonework blackened by years of smoke from the chimneys of woollen mills in this northern industrial town. I heard footsteps approaching and the door was opened by a maid in black and white uniform.

"Yes?"

"I'm Nurse Baines and I'm starting my training this morning."

"Midwifery?"

"No, district nursing."

At that moment a plump girl with short fair hair and a red face came gasping up the drive.

"Sorry I'm late."

"Midwifery?" queried the maid again.

"Yes, I am Sue Wiggins, I have to report to Miss Barker."

"Come in." The maid opened the door wider, then turning to me – "We're not expecting you but you'd better come in, I suppose."

The would-be midwife was bustled off to an office on the left, and I was asked to wait in the hall. The house was stunning of its time, typical of the many in the area that were built by the mill owners of the eighteenth and nineteenth centuries. There was a very wide sweeping staircase with a curved mahogany banister. Many of these houses were now used as public buildings since the decline of the textile trade in the early part of the twentieth century, and this one had been taken over by the Hatfield Borough Council District Nursing Service.

"Well now Nurse Baines," a very large lady in a navy blue suit descended on me, "I'm Miss Varley, we thought you were starting next week." She managed to imply it was my fault. "I'll introduce you to the district nurses and then we'll find you a uniform."

She took me into a large room filled with a long wooden table and cupboards all round. There were about ten nurses in outdoor uniforms of heavy gabardine coats and felt hats. The noise was indescribable as they were all arguing

"Why can't you go to Horley? – it's nearer to your area!"

"Don't give me that miserable complaining old beggar! I've got fifteen this morning, and then evening visits. I'm not taking any more!"

"Nurses! Nurses!" Miss Varley banged on the table with a stainless steel dish "This is Nurse Baines – she is starting her training with us today. Can somebody volunteer to take her round?"

There was a sullen silence while ten pairs of eyes looked at me with hostility.

Miss Varley pursed her lips "Very well Miss Grey, you will take Nurse Baines." She looked at a cross-faced woman of about fifty five.

"Aw! Why do I have to, Miss Varley? – I'm trying to cover Sister Walters' holidays!"

"Then you'll have plenty to show her won't you?"

Miss Varley was already marching off with me scuttling in pursuit.

"Oh bloody hell!" We heard Sister Grey's raised voice as we headed to the stairs. I had never come across this attitude before. During my SRN training there was always an unwritten rule of being willing to go the extra mile.

I followed Miss Varley to a bedroom where large cupboards were full of spare uniforms.

"Goodness you are small and thin." I was at fault again. She held up a tent of a dress. "This is the smallest I have I'm afraid – get changed and I'll be back in a minute." She passed me a blue dress with a starched white collar and cuffs. It dropped over my head almost to the floor and was at least three sizes too big.

"I can't possibly wear this, I look ridiculous!" I cried as she appeared again carrying an outdoor coat and hat.

"Nonsense nurse, it just needs a belt to tuck it up a bit." She fastened a belt around my waist and pulling the dress up, tucked it under the belt. Next came the coat, which was so oversized and heavy I nearly collapsed under its weight. The round felt hat with large brim was plonked on my head, where it settled just above my eyes.

"Well I'm certainly not wearing this hat! I can't see!" The horror of the situation was giving me courage to be defiant. Miss Varley looked at her handiwork and ignored my protests.

"A little cotton wool, I think," she said as she pushed it under the rim of the hideous hat to fix it above eye level.

"Now off you go – Sister Grey is waiting." I staggered towards the top of the beautiful staircase, where I descended, with voluminous coat billowing out like Scarlett O'Hara in Gone With the Wind; Sister Grey stood at the bottom staring in disbelief.

"Oh! – don't you look a bugger! – anyway, come on, we're late."

I scuttled miserably after her as fast as my oversized garb would allow. We crossed a cobbled yard to what had been a coach house in the mansion's heyday, and was now a large garage, full of little black A40 cars. We squeezed into one and she tossed her Gladstone bag onto the back seat.

We drove for about fifteen minutes in silence, weaving in and out through the traffic in town; finally chugging up an enormous hill, which gave me the feeling we would never make it, and at any minute would roll back down to the bottom again.

Pulling on the handbrake outside a row of very small old cottages, she snapped, "Now, keep up with me –

4

we're late!" and with that, she opened her door and shot down the path in one fluid movement and disappeared, whilst I struggled just to open my door. She had vanished but spotting an open door, I ventured in. The room was dark and dingy, full of heavy brown furniture. There was a very dirty window with the remnants of a holey lace curtain hanging on a nail.

The cold ashes of yesterday's fire were in the grate. The floor was covered in brown lino with holes everywhere and in the middle was what had been a multi-coloured peg rug. To the left of the fireplace was an ancient shallow brown sink, and to the right was a metal frame bed with a wizened old man sitting up in a nightshirt, with a woollen cap on his head.

"Good Morning Mr. Kershaw." Sister Grey was taking her coat off.

"Oh its you, you owd rat bag! What 'av you come for?"

"Now Mr. Kershaw, it's Monday morning, I have come to give you your injection and a bed bath."

"Well, I'm not 'aving a bath, it's t' cold to tek me clothes off!"

Sister Grey walked over to the bed and seized Mr. Kershaw by the front of his nightshirt and shook him from side to side.

"We've come to give you a bed bath and a bed bath you will have!"

I stood rooted to the spot in horror. I couldn't do this. I would go back to Miss Varley and tell her I'd changed my mind. I was used to clean hospital patients, whom we respected and who respected us. Mentally I rang matron at my old training hospital and asked her to take me back. I would do permanents nights, anything, but not this.

"Don't just stand there!" snapped Sister Grey, "take your coat off, fold it inside out and put it on a newspaper." Reluctantly I disrobed and put the heavy coat on top of hers, then we stripped Mr. Kershaw, taking care to keep him wrapped in warm blankets as much as possible as the room was cold and damp. When the kettle had boiled, we washed his scrawny body and put him in clean clothes.

"We'll see you again on Thursday to put another dressing on your foot," said Sister Grey, as we headed for the door.

"Goodbye, Mr. Kershaw." I smiled at him.

"Bugger off!" came the reply as a shoe whistled past my ear.

"Why do we put our coats on newspaper?" I asked, back in the car.

"Fleas!" came the monosyllabic reply.

Conditions at the next house were somewhat cleaner, and the patient less hostile, but we were set upon by two snappy mongrels. I watched Sister Grey in awe as she managed to kick one in the teeth with her right foot and the other with the left as they shot off yowling.

"How did you manage that?" I asked.

"Many years of practice – now hurry up."

And so the nightmare wore on. Dirty houses, scruffy bad tempered patients, working in dark, cold basement rooms, outside lavatories, snarling dogs, and newspaper to put our clothes on, newspaper to wrap dirty dressings in and put our bags on, and if asked what I should use for this or that, the answer was always "newspaper." The plastic bag had not yet made its entrance into district nursing, in fact nothing that could be classed as progress had. It was all, at least here in Hatfield, still in the dark ages.

To carry out sterile dressings we boiled instruments and tubes, some of them unrecognizable to me, in saucepans. The dressings themselves were handmade by the nurses using gauze and cotton wool and gamgee, a sort of mixture of the two, then put in a biscuit tin and baked in the oven. We had to trust the patients to do this for us. No theatre autoclaves to do it as in hospital.

Occasionally a patient or relative was pleased to see us, which in a way could be worse, as we were presented with a cup of tea, often in a greasy jam-jar. Sister Grey didn't bat an eyelid and down it went.

Back at the car two urchins were sitting on the bonnet.

"Give us a ride nurse! – give us a ride!" they pleaded.

Sister Grey completely ignored them and as we set off they slid into the gutter. We headed across town to do Sister Walters' "posh lot" and I soon found myself in a different world of wide tree-lined avenues and enormous properties from different periods.

"Now I'm going to drop you off and you can do three visits – here are the addresses." She gave me the instructions on a notepad.

"One is a simple re-bandage of a leg, and the other two are vitamin B injections. I'll pick you up again here in thirty minutes. I set off with a Gladstone bag she had given me and found the first patient and all went well, except that the skies had opened and rain was coming down very heavily. By the time I had found the second one I was soaked. However, I pressed on and was soon ringing the bell at the third patient's imposing door. It was opened by a very rakish looking man of about forty-five who, looking me up and down, ushered me into a hall full of antiques.

"Oh, I say," he said in a sexy public school voice, "you are <u>awfully</u> wet, aren't you?" He led me into an elegant sitting room, which had an inviting looking log fire crackling in the grate.

"Come and take all your wet clothes off, and I'll bring you a warm towel." His eyes travelled up and down my body, as he reached for my coat. I backed towards the staircase.

"Is my patient upstairs?" I managed to ask.

"Third door on the left dear, I will have the towel ready." He winked at me!

I gave the injection to a sweet old lady I found upstairs, hoping she was the patient. As I crept down again I heard him call out from the kitchen. "I'm bringing some tea!." I shot through the door and down the path.

"Everything okay?" Sister Grey asked as I climbed into the waiting car. "Fine" I said, deciding not to mention the sex maniac. I doubt he'd have asked Sister Grey to take her clothes off.

We rattled over cobblestones up another enormous hill. These cobbles dated from when horses had pulled heavy carts up the hills and had been essential for the horses to keep their feet. We visited the last two patients and it was one pm. I had to be back at the nurses' home for lunch. Sister Grey was going home. To my disgust, she dropped me at a bus stop about two miles out of town.

For the first time I had the opportunity to look down upon the town I had come to train in. A pall of smokey grime hung over the valley. The stone buildings were blackened with many years of industrial pollution. There were huge mills and mill chimneys visible through the smog, although their heyday past, many were now disused. Two large gasometers vied with electricity cooling towers for the prize of ugliest structure. I gazed across the town I had agreed to work in for eighteen months and wondered how I would possibly stick it.

In front of me at the bus stop was a young mother with a little boy about six years old. They were giving me some very funny looks and I became aware again how ridiculous I looked in this ill fitting uniform and hat, now droopy and wet and sliding down over my eyes again. Gradually, more people came along and joined the queue. The little boy climbed on the rail of the bus stop, never taking his eyes off the strange apparition that was me. Then he put his legs over the rail and hung upside down to see if I looked any better that way up. Finally he spoke loud enough for all to hear.

"Mummy – is that a person?"

* * * * *

Once more, I hurried up the path of the nurses' home aware I was late for lunch and again, with much huffing and puffing, the little fat midwife caught me up.

"Oh! – I've had such an awful morning" she gasped, "I'm exhausted and I'm starving, and they're all barmy here, they're obsessed with newspaper! My name is Sue by the way."

"Pam, how do you do? You can't have had a worse morning than me – and I know all about the newspaper."

"I did my first home delivery." Sue was doing second part midwifery following six months training in hospital. She was qualified to deliver babies under supervision.

"Don't tell me you've had to wrap the baby in newspaper?"

"No, but what do you think I've got in here?" She held out a large newspaper parcel.

"Fish and chips?"

"It's the placenta! We have to bring them back here to go in the incinerator. I've had to carry it on the bus."

We dashed in, washed our hands and presented ourselves in the dining room, being scolded for lateness. As I started to eat a delicious hot meal Miss Varley appeared at my side.

"I don't want you to work this afternoon Nurse. We are short for the evening shift. Finish your lunch and come back on duty at six pm. Your new uniform will be here in a few days by the way."

I opened my mouth to say 'please don't bother, I'm leaving just as soon as I've eaten this.' – but somehow the words didn't come out. I couldn't be as feeble as to let it beat me. I would give it a week, then review the situation.

I presented myself at the duty room at five-fifty pm. Three other sisters were there arguing about the evening visits. A rather large mature lady with a strong Irish accent was telling them she couldn't take the heavy ones as her back was bad.

"Ah – Sister O'Neill. I've done something about that." Miss Varley came into the room. "Nurse Baines is going around with you so you can take most of the heavies – she'll help you with the lifting."

Sister O'Neill shot me a look of pure hatred. After a further exchange of angry unpleasantries, we set off in the direction of the garage. As soon as we opened the door, Sister O'Neill crossed herself.

"Holy Mary – Mother of God – will you look at the fog!"

She was right. We had to almost grope to the cars. Not only was it dark, but a thick damp industrial fog enveloped us.

Clutching the steering wheel, she set off with her nose almost pressed on the windscreen.

"We've got six visits and we'll still be going round at midnight so we will," she said as we edged out into the main road to the tune of car horns from all sides. As we climbed up out of the town visibility improved and our spirits rose as we got through four visits – a penicillin injection and three very ill patients to make comfortable.

Underneath her brusque manner Sister O'Neill was kind and caring, and it was obvious how much the patients and relatives appreciated us. I was almost beginning to enjoy myself. This was not to last. As we dropped down the hillside the fog met us again, this time twice as thick.

"I want you to stick your head out and look for Cameron Road, it's here somewhere on the left."

We crept along hugging the pavement, which was barely visible until suddenly Sister O'Neill thought she saw a turning. As she swung her wheel left, we started bouncing manically up and down. Our heads bumped on the roof, and as we tried to cling on to the doors a horrible grinding sound came from under the car – we had driven down a flight of steps! The car stalled and slid to a halt as we hit the road at the bottom, a St Christopher medal swinging wildly from the rear view mirror. Where were you when we needed you? I thought.

Somehow, we pulled ourselves together, and amazingly the car seemed little the worse for our adventure. We attended our penultimate patient before crawling off again to find the last visit with Sister O'Neill calling frequently on the Holy Mother to give us some divine intervention.

This time we really did seem to be going round in circles. The road was strangely narrow and all the other traffic had disappeared. The light from our headlamps reflected back at us from the damp grey blanket of fog. It was nearly ten o'clock and I was exhausted and felt this ghastly day would never end. Suddenly, we spotted a small sign at the left hand side. Sister dug me in the ribs. "Get out and see if it says Akers Road, please Holy Mary, let it be!" We both crossed ourselves.

I bent over the sign in the gloom, then climbed back into the car.

"Well, does it say it Akers road girl?"

"Nope! It says "Please keep off the grass!" We were driving round the park.

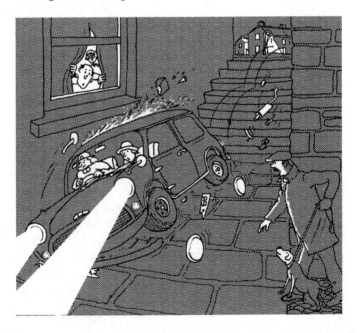

Chapter 2

At the end of the first week, I took stock. My training period was to be six months, followed by an exam. After this, I was supposed to work a further twelve months as a duty to my employing authority for going to the trouble of training me. I was to carry out this work on foot in all weathers, except when I could use my bus pass, in the unlikely event I could find a bus going anywhere near my next patient.

I hated the poverty, the scruffy dirty streets and houses, the mostly ungrateful patients, the snarling dogs, and the grimy depressing atmosphere in the town. I felt I had stepped back in time a hundred years.

However, I knew that once qualified, I could take a post in a much more pleasant area, getting around by car. I had married just before I started my district training and we lived about five miles away in a pretty semi-rural village.

So I decided to stick it out and with grim determination I buckled down. There were four others on the training course and we got on well, comparing notes and sharing experiences, most of them hilarious. We had one study day per week when Miss Varley gave us lectures. We learned about all the services which were available to our patients such as home helps, meals on wheels, chiropody, and how to liaise with hospitals and GPs. We learned how to take our hospital skills out into the community, and how to nurse patients with various conditions in the home.

As far as nursing aids were concerned we were taught to adapt common or garden household items as necessary, for example, if a bed-cradle was needed to take the weight of the bedclothes off the patient's legs why not use a fireguard? We found this ridiculous – why couldn't we have our own supply of equipment? This was to come of course, but was still a revolutionary idea to the likes of Miss Varley and her ilk. She really excelled herself when showing us how to boil our instruments in a saucepan to sterilize them.

"And should the pans you are given be very stained nurses, boiling a stick of rhubarb in them will remove all the stains."

We were shown how to fold newspaper into a bag for this and a receptacle for that and always to put our coats and bags on to this wonderful ubiquitous stuff.

After surviving the first month and getting to know the ropes, we began to feel that we might just make it. We hadn't reckoned on the weather.

The winter of 1962-63 was to become known as the "big freeze" and easily able to give 1947 a run for its money, never to be forgotten by anyone whose job involved travelling around in the great outdoors. The snow started to fall in January and was to continue on and off until the end of April, but without any thaw to get rid of what had already fallen. As the council workmen tried to keep the roads clear huge frozen mounds of snow built up at the sides of roads and paths.

Bus timetables meant nothing as public transport arrived sporadically, if at all. The temperature was so arctic that waiting at a bus stop meant freezing to death became a distinct possibility. We soon developed an almost permanent state of exhaustion struggling around in the cold, trying to wade through snowdrifts up to our knickers. I took to wearing long woolly ones and woolly vests.

The patients seemed oblivious to the drama going on outside.

"By, you're late this morning, what time you do call this?" was a common reaction to the front door opening and a snowman-like district nurse falling in.

Having got the patient up, I would gaze longingly at the bed and want to crawl into it myself, a feeling I hadn't had since my last night duty, when I had worked fifteen nights non-stop during a flu epidemic. On the worst days when snow fell heavily we took to begging lifts on anything still moving. Farmers with tractors were favourites as they definitely kept going, but we usually smelled a little ripe when we jumped off.

Waiting in vain at a bus stop one morning I accepted an offer of a lift from a lecherous looking type with snow chains on the wheels of his sports car. He kept stroking my nearest leg, but past caring, it seemed a small price to pay to get back to the nurses' home and a hot meal.

Evening visits were a nightmare but at least we went in twos in the car, with a bag of sand and two shovels in the boot. The snow driving skills of the drivers varied, but the steep hills in every direction would test the abilities of an alpine rally ace. I found it quite comforting to cross myself like Sister O'Neill as we frequently sailed round in three hundred and sixty degree turns, before becoming embedded in a six-foot snowdrift, but we soon dug ourselves out and carried on until the next drama. This was to prove excellent training for the years ahead.

* * *

As part of our training we had to spend one day with a health visitor and one with a midwife. The health visitor came first and I was allocated to Miss Johnson. She was a kind lady nearing retirement and was dressed quite severely in a dark Harris tweed suit with flat lace-up shoes and a navy hat. This was how a health visitor was expected to dress and the younger ones coming into the job hated looking so dowdy and old-fashioned, and loathed wearing hats in particular.

The emphasis of health visiting was on child care and advice, but they would also advise on all aspects of health and welfare in the home. It was their statutory duty to take over from the midwife when the baby was ten days old. They were responsible for running child welfare clinics and vaccination and immunization programmes. The doctor present at these clinics was either the medical officer of health or one of his deputies.

Miss Johnson met me in her Morris Minor at the nurses' home.

"Come along dear, we have a lot to get through." She looked rather harassed.

Driving carefully and peeping out from behind horn-rimmed spectacles she looked a bit like an owl. I asked her to tell me about her training and was interested to hear she had done her S.R.N at Guy's Hospital in London in the nineteen twenties, had done her midwifery in Liverpool in the nineteen thirties and her health visiting back in Yorkshire, where she had come from. I asked her if she had been happy nursing.

"Oh yes dear, most of the time – but on a bad day I sometimes wish I had married instead."

I found it very sad that up until the late forties nurses who married had to leave the profession. It was felt by the matrons of the day, most of whom had been left on the shelf, that nurses who married could not be totally committed to their patients.

The ward sisters and sister tutors who had trained me had all been unmarried. They had often had to make a terrible choice and many must have regretted their decision to dedicate their lives to nursing when they found themselves facing a lonely and childless old age. Miss Johnson had been secretly engaged to young doctor in her days as a staff nurse at Guy's, but had loved her job so much she had decided to choose her career instead. He had married another nurse some time later and had had an illustrious career and been knighted for his pioneering work in eye surgery.

Our first visit of the day was on a large council estate known for its lawlessness and where many of the inhabitants regularly spent Saturday nights in casualty after drunken brawls and wife beating.

"They're not bad people really dear, they just don't know any better," said Miss Johnson.

I didn't know if I would be able to feel so benevolent towards them. Our first mother had just had her ninth child. Some were white, whilst others were brown with tight curly hair. Whilst Miss Johnson examined the baby the others were running wild in bare feet and various stages of half dress. One little boy was wearing a torn woolly jumper with a bare bottom, while the next one down the pecking order sported some short pants but no top. A little girl of about four years wore a nightdress and watched us from the corner of the room whilst cramming what looked like dry bread into her mouth, which she was sharing with the dog. Three older children were squabbling in the kitchen.

"Shouldn't the children be at school today Mary?" Miss Johnson enquired.

"Well they 'avent no shoes, the social don't give me enough to clothe this lot – I keep telling you that." The hard-faced mother was only twenty nine but she looked about fifty. A cigarette dangled from her mouth and some ash dropped onto the baby's face.

"I thought the W.R.V.S. brought you some shoes last week," Miss Johnson persisted, "what happened to those?"

"'Ere," said the mother beginning to look aggressive, "don't come in 'ere telling me how to look after me kids! I bet you 'aven't any!" This was a frequent retort Miss Johnson was to explain, and if things weren't kept amicable they would refuse to let the health visitors in at all. It was like walking on egg shells.

"Of course the husband or boyfriend of the moment often takes the shoes or clothes that we give them to the pub and sells them. What can we do? It's so hard to help the children. They are deprived and are growing up to be the delinquents of tomorrow."

We drove to a shabby terraced row back in town for our next visit which was to an Asian family. Immigrants from India and Pakistan had been flooding in to the north of England over the last few years mainly because of the textile industry.

"The problem here will be communication; so few of them speak English to any degree, particularly the women who lead such cloistered lives at home," Miss Johnson explained and said she had been asked to call by a G.P. concerned about a goat being kept in the back yard!

"Oh it often happens but their culture is so different to ours, keeping livestock to them is normal."

We entered by the back yard and saw the goat tethered in the coal place which had no door. It was happily eating some cabbage leaves and its droppings were very much in evidence as we picked our way across the yard. In the kitchen a young Asian lady was making chapattis on the floor, and several other women were sitting round in the front room. There wasn't a man in sight which was a shame as they would have had some rudimentary English as Miss Johnson had no success at all with the ladies who stared at us silently.

"I shall have to report it to the sanitation department and they can deal with it," said Miss Johnson as we climbed back in the car. The morning flew past until our last visit before going for lunch. This was to a young mother who had two children, one eighteen months old and one six months.

It was obvious as she let us in that she wasn't pleased to see us.

"I'm concerned that you haven't brought the babies for their immunizations yet Sharon" said Miss Johnson, picking up the toddler who was busy trying to poke something into an electric socket.

"No and I'm not going to do neither. I told you last time we don't believe in it."

Miss Johnson explained again how safe vaccination was and how nasty, and even fatal, some of the childhood diseases could be.

"Well my mum says just as many kids are ill after the jabs as what it prevents, she says they don't tell us the half, that it's all hushed up, and my husband's little brother Alfie went cross-eyed after his smallpox so he says I haven't to take them, so you can just piss off!"

Miss Johnson suddenly looked weary. She patted the little ones and said good-bye to Sharon without another word.

"In the face of such determined ignorance what can we do?" she sighed as we got back into the car.

In the afternoon we drove to one of the outlying villages to an old Methodist Sunday school building next to the chapel. This was used every Monday afternoon for a baby clinic. A circle of mums sat holding naked babies wrapped in towels. Some of the babies were blissfully asleep and some were bawling their heads off. A member of the clerical staff from the health department sat at a table selling tins of baby food, and concentrated orange juice and cod liver oil were given out free of charge.

In the examination room we both put white coats on and I was introduced to a very pleasant lady doctor who was going to examine all the first visit babies and any that Miss Johnson or a mum was worried about.

Two of the conditions babies were screened for in the early months were congenital displacement of the hip joints and cystic fibrosis, a nasty condition of the lungs and digestive system which was fatal but had a much better prognosis if diagnosed early.All the babies were weighed and their progress or lack of it was monitored. They were then given whatever vaccinations were due.

Quite a few of the babies had nappy rash and Miss Johnson handed out cream and advice as necessary.

At least half of the mothers were breast feeding which pleased Miss Johnson and the doctor. "It can be difficult to persuade some of them to try but a lot of these mums are quite hard up and apart from being much better for the babies it's much cheaper. Sometimes we even have to encourage them to wean the children off the breast especially when the next baby is on the way."

She told me about one mum in Liverpool when she trained who was still breast feeding her four year old little boy. He would just lift her jumper and help himself anytime, anywhere. Neighbours were free with their advice, – 'paint a scary face on your boobs', he loved them and brought all his friends in for a look, 'paint bitter aloes on your nipples' – he loved that too!

"What happened in the end?" I was dying to know.

"Oh I've no idea – he's probably still at it."

* * *

My day with the midwife came the following week and I met Sister Warley at the nurses' home at eight thirty a.m. She was a down to earth, no nonsense Yorkshire woman of the type you'd want on your side in an emergency.

Our first visit was to the Asian area of the town. As immigrants they tended to flock together and as houses came up for sale whole streets became populated by Asians. However Indians and Pakistanis had no time for each other. A caste system operated with Pakistanis regarded as inferior by the Indians.

Our patient was a young Pakistani woman who had started in labour in the early hours of the morning.

Asian women often had to have their babies in hospital as they tended to have low birth weight babies needing an incubator and special baby care. Another reason for hospital delivery was poor or unclean home circumstances. Often English mothers having their first babies couldn't get a bed in hospital and this caused some resentment.

However this patient was having her third child and was regarded as suitable for home delivery. Arriving at the bedside we found our labouring patient was having to share her bed with a very old lady who was happily snoring her head off.

Sister Warley was having none of that. She woke the old woman and mimed "get out of the bed and buzz off, quick sharp!" The old lady babbled something in Urdu and turning over tried to ignore us, where upon Sister grabbed her and pulling her out of bed, pushed her out of the room. In the middle of this power struggle the patient was making terrible ear splitting howls with every contraction. Sister Warley decided she needed to examine her internally and sent me downstairs to ask for a bowl of hot water and a clean towel. This proved easier said than done as I was met with the usual blank stare.

"Bowl? bowl? towel?" I asked as I mimed hand washing and drying. No result. In desperation I opened a cupboard and found an enamel bowl which I pounced upon. I pointed at the kettle and said "Water – hot water." But meanwhile the old lady we had dragged from the arms of Morpheus had grabbed the other side of the bowl to wrest it from my grasp, and an unseemly struggle followed which I won hands down, and dashing upstairs with my trophy told Sister water was to follow. Behind me came three of the ladies each carrying a cup full of water and eventually, after many more journeys, we had a decent bowl of water. Sister decided progress was satisfactory, if slow, and we would return later in the day.

Calling into the nurses' home Sister received a message to meet an ambulance on Boot street to attend a spontaneous abortion. This was the street where local prostitutes plied their trade. A few minutes later we pulled up behind the ambulance which was outside a block of toilets.

"Glad to see you love," said one of the ambulance men to Sister Warley. The patient was sitting moaning on one of the toilets refusing to go with the ambulance men. Her friend, dressed in black fishnet tights and five inch high heels, a tiny mini skirt and a boob tube told us our patient had taken two packets of Carters little liver pills to make sure she 'got rid'. It was a sordid little scene but without turning a hair Sister W had her off the toilet and in the ambulance in no time.She sighed as they left. "It's easy to look down our noses at these girls, but they've come from poor homes where their mothers probably did the same thing, so we ought to think there but for the Grace of God."

We visited several new mothers and babies at home as they were the district midwifes' responsibility for the first ten days post natal. One visit to a new mum whose baby had died a few hours after delivery was very sad and Sister Warley spent quite some time talking to her and trying to console her.

Next it was back to our Asian labouring mum to check on progress where the first job was to haul the old lady out of bed again. She let us have it with a mouthful of Urdu which was probably an ancient curse.

"And the same to you madam!" said Sister W as she disappeared down the stairs. We tried to reassure our patient we would be back soon as really not much was happening.

After lunch it was off to an ante natal clinic. The personal hygiene of a few of the patients left a lot to be desired. Sister Warley had to bend down over the patient's abdomen, to listen to the baby's heart beat, with her nose next to the genital area.

"Sharon dear, when did you last have a bath?" she enquired of one young lady.

"Ooh, me mum says you shouldn't have a bath when you're expecting! I haven't had one for six months, and I haven't washed me hair neither!"

Sister quietly explained that her mother was quite wrong and suggested that she should have a bath every day. Sharon left looking doubtful.

We finished the ante-natal clinic in time for a quick cup of tea before it was back to our Asian lady.

"What do you bet the old crone will be back in the bed?" I asked.

"Surely, she wouldn't dare." said Sister Warley. But there she was and the usual curses were cast upon us. An hour and a half later the baby was about to be born. Mum was pushing amid much wailing and shouting in Urdu. I was administering gas and air at the top end as Sister W was working at the bottom. Suddenly a door in the corner of the room, which I had assumed to be a cupboard, opened and at least eight Asian men walked nonchalently through the room. "Who are they? – where have they come from?" I gasped in astonishment.

"It's the night shift going to work," Sister was not thrown off her stride in any way, "they've been asleep in the attic all day and if we're here much longer the day shift will walk through going to bed! – Come on Mum, push! <u>Push!</u>"

Finally we delivered a beautiful baby boy. "Thank the Lord he's healthy and in one piece, I always give a prayer of thanks these days" said Sister Warley.

Midwives all over the country were coming to the end of a distressing time of delivering deformed babies. A drug named thalidomide, developed in Germany, mainly for calming elderly patients had unfortunately been given to pregnant mums to help with sleep problems for several years before it was noticed that it was causing neo-natal deformities and many babies were born with arms or legs missing or just present as stumps.

When the cause was identified and the drug taken off the market, the last babies which could possibly be affected were born in August 1962. A dreadful time was over for the doctors and midwives but a lifetime of struggle for many was just beginning. The legal case against the makers of the drug dragged on for many years with compensation finally being paid.

Sister W said she had delivered one terribly deformed little boy and her next delivery had been a beautiful healthy little girl whose mother had grumbled because she had wanted a boy. "It was all I could do not to say come with me , I'll show you a little boy!"

It was going dark as we arrived back at the nurses' home ready to go off duty. For Sister Warley it was not to be. The Midwifery Superintendent was waiting for her.

"It's Nellie I'm afraid. Sister Green's out on a call and Sister Smith has rung in with flu. I'll have to ask you to go," she turned to me, "Nurse Baines you can go off duty."

I looked at a very weary Sister Warley. "I'll come with you if you think I can help," I offered, "who's Nellie anyway?"

"Nellie is about to have baby number thirteen, and has refused point blank to go into hospital," said Sister as we collected extra equipment and headed back in to town.

The guidelines from the Department of Health was now that primips – women having their first babies – and grand multigravidas – women who had had multiple births should be encouraged to give birth in hospital as figures showed this was much safer, but if a mother refused she had to be supported at home by the district midwives.

We were heading towards the older part of town where much of the housing had been condemned and in the not too distant future would be demolished, the occupants to be scattered round various large estates of council housing. Nellie's small house was in a court. These small squares of housing were a relic of industrial Britain, with many of the houses closed in and getting little sunlight and fresh air.

We parked and collecting bags and sheets went into Raglan Court. It was like stepping back into Dickens' time. The water was taken from a tap in the court shared by about ten homes. Slops were thrown out on to the flagstones and drained away in a gulley along its' length. At the back of the houses was another yard containing outside privies which again were shared by several families.

We found Nellie groaning with her labour pains on a settee in the kitchen. Everybody else had gone to bed and left her to it. My first job was to fill the sooty old kettle from the tap in the yard and put it on the two ring gas appliance and find a bucket to empty the water into every time Sister needed to wash her hands to examine Nellie, to check on her progress which by now was speeding up.

Emptying the bucket into the sink, I found my legs and feet soaked – the sink was not connected to the drain!

Nellie looked at me in disgust. "Have you no sense?" How silly of me to expect the sink to be connected. Half an hour later I set off into the back yard with a small torch to find the privy, clutching my bucket. A small building loomed up in the dark and the smell told me what it was.

I tried to stand as far back as I could, and just as I was about to let fly with the bucket, I heard a noise behind me and felt hot breath on my neck. Almost paralyzed with terror I turned and found myself eyeball to eyeball with a horse! He nuzzled and pushed at me until I was trapped in the offensively foul smelling privy. Enjoying a bit of company in his lonely night, he stood blocking any hope of escape. I heard Sister Warley calling my name and in desperation, still clutching my bucket, I ducked under the horse and got back into the house.

Sister looked up from Nellie's nether regions. "The baby's nearly here!"

"Never mind the baby! Nellie, did you know there's a horse in the yard?"

Nellie stopped pushing and put on her poshest voice. "Hof course I know there's a 'orse in the yard. My 'usband's a rag and bone man."

Number thirteen popped out with no problem just as we heard a horrible scratching and scuttering in the corner near our coats.

"What was that? Nellie, have you got mice?" asked Sister Warley.

"No, but next door are a right mucky lot," said Nellie, "and their rats come up our drain."

Dawn was breaking as we left Nellie and her baby, the horse and the rats. It was all grist to the mill.

* * *

"I wouldn't be in your shoes!" One of the sisters looked at me with a strangely pitying expression as I came into the duty room to do evening visits. Damn! What had I done now?

"Ah – nurse Baines." Miss Varley was wearing her 'let's look on the brighter side' expression.

"You have your usual list tonight plus two new patients; a Mr Wilson on Cardigan Street with pneumonia and er," she coughed and cleared her throat, "a Mrs Heggarty on Pellon Lane – spontaneous abortion for penicillin injections."

I was aware of the silence and all eyes were on me, but I hadn't a clue why.

"Go on then – what's the joke?"

"Haven't you heard of the Heggartys?" Sister Smith looked amazed.

"Are they famous then?"

"Infamous – half of them get locked up for drunken brawling every Saturday night. The police will only go down their street in twos."

Sister Fawcett put in her two pen'orth, "and the last time the hire purchase man called they threw him through the window into the gutter!"

There was nothing I could do about it. They lived bang in the middle of my area. They were my patients.

28

We all set off together, the walkers cadging lifts from the drivers. I tried to keep my mind off the heinous Heggartys as I worked steadily through my patients until I had to head in their direction for my last visit.

I could see which house it was without counting numbers. Dull brown paint was peeling off the windows and doors. Raggy, grey net curtains covered the glass. Rain dripped from a broken guttering down the wall and weeds had managed to gain a footing on both sides of the door. There was a note hanging from a nail on the front door. Maybe it was for me and my patient had gone into hospital! It said "RENT MAN – f— off or you'll get it" I didn't think they meant the rent. I banged the door knocker and heard a large vicious sounding dog snarling and barking somewhere at the other side. The door was opened by a slight young man with blue eyes and dark hair, in his twenties. He was clean and tidy and didn't look too alarming.

"Ah Sister! – please will you come in?" He had a soft Irish accent.

I stepped onto bare boards; the house was cold. He led me upstairs; more bare boards and an empty packing crate for a bedside table. My patient, looking pale and sad, lay on a mattress on the floor covered by a rough blanket and two overcoats. On the packing crate was a tray laid with a clean white cloth, a small bowl, a new tablet of soap and a clean towel.

"I'll bring some hot water for you to wash your hands and may I take your coat Sister?"

Mary wept quietly as she told me this would have been their first baby – no procured abortion this.

As I finished the injection and tried to comfort her, Mr Heggarty cuddled his wife.

29

"Can I make you a cup of tea Sister, sure we're very grateful to you for coming?"

Politely declining, I told them I'd see them tomorrow and I hoped Mary would be able to sleep. A priest was on the doorstep as I was leaving. Mr Heggarty introduced us and we shook hands. As I left, Father O'Malley was offering condolences about the baby.

Nothing very exciting to tell them in the duty room after all.

* * *

As the snow finally melted, our exam drew nearer. We all felt ill prepared as we'd been too tired to swot and whilst out there like Scott of the Antarctic, the exam had seemed the least of our worries. As panic set in, we asked each other questions like "How do you apply for a compulsory removal order? – is it one magistrate or two?"

"Don't worry yer heads," said Sister O'Neill, "Ye'll never get one – I've given up trying." In truth it wasn't the written papers we were worried about, it was the practical exam. Practicals were always harrowing, working with real patients, being observed by an invariably sour faced Sister tutor examiner.

"Have ye heard who's coming to do your practical?" asked Sister O'Neill.

"Her name's Miss Healey."

"Holy Mary! – Mother o'God – is that auld witch still going round?" she crossed herself vigorously.

Miss Healey arrived on the following Monday to stay in the nurses' home for the exam week, and the day of my practical dawned. She marched out to her car with me trotting behind carrying my bag. She was a large lady with a marked resemblance to a well known comedian in drag. Her car was the traditional Morris Minor which she drove with eyes staring fixedly ahead, her enormous feet planted on the pedals with her plump black stockinged legs wide apart occasionally showing flashes of long pink bloomers.

She didn't speak and apart from giving directions I had the sense to remain silent unless spoken to. She roared along, mostly in second gear, ignoring stop signs and everybody else's right of way, completely oblivious to the chaos left in her wake.

I had spent weeks getting my selection of patients prepared. Everything had to be "a la text book" to the nth degree, which meant a lot of pallavouring about with masses of sheets, towels, buckets and bowls, bed pans, hot water, jugs, instruments and lotions, dressings, plaster, plaster remover, rubber gloves, tubes and newspaper, newspaper, newspaper; and most importantly making it look as if we always did it like that. The trouble was she knew we didn't and we knew she knew we didn't and so on.

Just in case she was in any doubt, my first patient, who had even put some newspaper round the light fitting, asked anxiously if she'd got everything right for me, as looking at Miss Healey, "we don't usually carry on like this." The old witch gave me a "ha ha – just as I thought," look and that was how it went on all morning. The blanket bath at old Mr Smith's was fine until he pinched my bottom as I tucked his sheet in and I cried out, "Oh Mr Smith! – not today," as if it was alright any other day.

The Cairn terrier at Balaclava Terrace took exception to Miss Healey's size eight feet and sank his teeth into her ankle as we were leaving. "You should have the animals under control Nurse!" she snapped. All hopes of passing had long since deserted me and as we headed back towards the nurses' home she launched into a diatribe about what a disgrace to the profession my generation of nurses was. Just at that time the Royal College of Nursing was becoming ever so slightly militant for the first time in history in an attempt to secure for us an increase in remuneration which might just lift us off the bread line.

"Disgraceful!" she shrieked, "nursing is a vocation, an honour, a privilege, how dare you demean us by bringing it down to the level of money? You ought to be ashamed of yourselves!"

One would have thought I alone had instigated the whole thing. She finished off, of all things, on the subject of underwear. "You silly young girls, with your flimsy modern underwear! No wonder the old men tweak your bottoms! Disgraceful! No one ever tweaked my bottom!"

At last I had something going for me. Following the bitter weather my woolly underwear was second to none. I lifted my uniform to show her my vest and long woolly knickers. She had difficulty believing her eyes but from that moment her attitude changed. I passed!

We all passed and became Queen's District Nursing Sisters. A certain William Rathbone had started a system providing visiting nurses for the poor in Liverpool in the late nineteenth century and had gained the patronage of Queen Victoria.

Before the beginning of the Health Service in 1948 many district nurses were paid for by public subscription. Local district nursing associations, affiliated to the Queen's Institute, employed these nurses, paying their salaries and expenses and usually providing houses or nurses' homes for them. When I thought of these early worthy ladies working in the slums, my admiration for them knew no bounds. I had worked for the last six months with poor families, in poor housing, and I was well aware I was seeing the last of these conditions.

Spring finally came and with it the thaw, but on the hills snow could be seen in the corners of the fields into the summer. Sue passed her second part midwifery and left for pastures new and we four newly qualified nurses looked forward to doing the same thing. Until then we carried on trudging up the hills and pounding the mean streets and getting soaked to the skin on a regular basis.

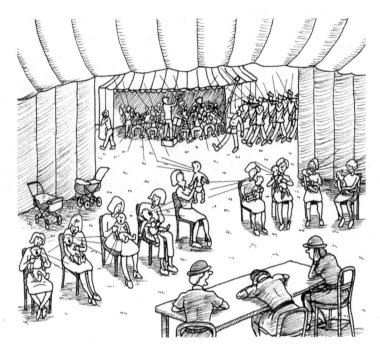

Chapter 3

Just before my year of working for my training authority was up, a job was advertised for a district nurse in the village where I lived. The area was partly rural and partly urban, having several villages situated around the small town of Bridgend. There was even a house with the job which was in a pretty area near the church. I could hardly believe my luck that the opportunity should come up just as I finished my training.

As a newly qualified and somewhat inexperienced applicant I daren't allow myself to get too excited but I was granted an interview with Dr Scrimshaw, medical officer of health for the Bridgend area and the Nurse Manager of district nurses, midwives and health visitors, Miss Burton.

Dr Scrimshaw the M.O.H was a rather effeminate bachelor of about fifty, who was known to hold some very eccentric views on all sorts of topics that were none of his business.

Whenever there was a shortage of local news the Bridgend Echo would ask him for a quote which would form the headline on the front page such as, "Medical Officer of Health says teenagers eat too many chips," or some such ludicrous pronouncement. Now he proceeded to ask me some very odd questions which seemed quite irrelevant to whether I was a good candidate for the job or not.

"Are you one of these modern young ladies who likes to listen to this pop music by the er – the er – Spiders?"

"I think you mean the Beatles Doctor," said the nursing officer.

"Yes I like the Beatles," I said thinking I must be in the wrong interview.

"Well I hope you don't wear mini skirts or paint your toe nails."

"Er – no."

"Tell me nurse, how do you feel about working mothers?" asked Miss Burton.

Oh God, let me out of here, I thought but before I could answer, the nutty doctor played his trump card.

"And are you able to have a cooked meal ready for your husband when you've been out all day looking after your patients?"

"Oh that's no problem; my oven switches itself on." I replied.

Well, it did but I'd never bothered to work out how to set it. Dr Scrimshaw slapped the desk with delight. "Did you hear that Miss Burton? What a sensible young lady!" And that was it, I got the job.

Following a short discussion about the house that was available with the job, Rob and I decided to stay where we were and no one seemed to mind either way.

My new job was very different in many ways from working in a large industrial town. No more trudging round on foot, frozen and soaked to the skin. My little second hand car, brought on hire purchase, felt like paradise. No more sharing out work with a bunch of bad tempered colleagues. I worked alone from my home with my telephone. The local doctors knew to call before nine a.m, or at lunch time with new visits, and messages were received from the Health Department or the hospitals. As long as I did the work to everybody's satisfaction I was able to come and go as I pleased.

Sometimes things were hectically busy and sometimes fairly quiet but the rough was taken with the smooth. The local doctors were very friendly and made me feel welcome and the local people – my patients – were delightful compared to the ungrateful lot I'd had in Hatfield.

For days off I worked with Edna the nurse who did the Queenstown area and we relieved each other. Queenstown was a very working class mill town, famous for its championship band attached to one of the mills. It was said that you could get a job there without any of the skills that were of use to the textile trade as long as you could play a brass instrument.

My area was much more middle class and Edna would say, "I wouldn't have your posh lot for all the tea in China kid, all they have to do to get you running round is pick up the phone."

Most of the Queenstown residents were not 'on the phone'. She was right that Queenstown folk were a more independent sort with a strong community spirit, where families pulled together and neighbours helped each other out.

Our employing authority was the West Riding of Yorkshire and we were division eighteen. There were three nurses working the Bridgend district and three more did Eastham and surrounding villages. Edna was firmly of the opinion that we should keep to ourselves, even if it meant missing an odd day off here and there, if one of us was on holiday. So no matter how busy we were, we coped alone.

"If we don't bother them they won't bother us kid," she would say, although it could be pretty hard going out every evening if we had evening visits and patients were often on twice daily penicillin injections.

Edna was pretty easy going as a work colleague but it soon became obvious she preferred animals to humans. She had had the benefit of a good education and had wanted to be a vet, but this was at a time when few women went to university and her Victorian parents thought it a quite ridiculous idea. They eventually agreed to allow her to train as a nurse at St James's Hospital in Leeds, but for Edna it was a poor substitute. She followed her general training with midwifery and then district nurse training. When she took the post at Queenstown, moving into the house provided, the patients soon worked out that she knew a lot about animals and their ailments and that it was cheaper to visit her than the vet. When visiting her patients I would quite often find the dog sporting a familiar N.H.S bandage, or the cat would run off with a yowl at the sight of my uniform.

I'd just finished giving Mrs Clark her insulin injection when she said, "Before you go I want you to look at the budgie." I glanced into the cage. The budgie stared gloomily back.

"He's very nice," I said.

"Yes but he's off his food. What do you think I should do about it?"

"I've no idea, Mrs Clark, I don't know anything about budgies." Mrs Clark looked quite miffed.

"Well that's no good, our proper nurse would know. When is she back?"

"Not till next week I'm afraid," I said, feeling inadequate.

"He might be dead by then!!" she called indignantly as I disappeared down the path.

The main doctors' surgery on my patch was a large three doctor practice. Drs Galbraith, Galbraith and Craig were Scots and the surgery was one room in Dr Galbraith senior's house. A waiting room had been built on at the back which had a bare asphalt floor and wooden benches for the patients to sit on. One elderly receptionist sat in another small room answering the telephone. In all respects it was the same as when Dr Galbraith had put up his brass plate just after the First World War, in which he had served at the front as a medical officer.

As I went round meeting my new patients, I could tell some were wary of my lack of experience due to my age.

"Have you done your training? You don't look old enough," I heard several times but I also heard old Dr

Galbraith was going round saying, "Och! she'll do fine – she's a grand wee lassie."

If I was alright for him, I'd do. I was accepted and my heart warmed to him.

He was a wonderful man; highly respected by the local people he had cared for for over forty years.

The other surgery on my district was run by a single handed G.P – Dr Smith. It too was a room in his home almost as old fashioned as the Galbraiths.

A lot of general practitioners were banding together to form group practices and building modern surgeries, but just as many still used rooms in their own homes and were not moving with the times.

Dr Scrimshaw, the medical officer who had given me the job, also lived on my patch with his elderly housekeeper and she became one of my first patients when Dr Craig rang me.

"Can you go and visit Pansy Potter's housekeeper? She's got a chest infection. Twice daily penicillin and general care."

"Who's Pansy Potter?"

"Your boss – Dr Scrimshaw, and take your sun glasses."

Dr Scrimshaw opened the door. Away from his office he appeared more eccentric than ever. His hair was wild and uncombed and he was wearing a baggy grey cardigan with holes in the elbows. He showed me into his sitting room which was a picture of muddle and chaos.

"I'm just writing my annual report. It's got to be at the printers on Monday – sit down, sit down."

I sat gingerly on a chair covered in papers. On every possible surface were papers and books and empty tea cups.

"I've lost chapter two," he muttered, "get up girl, get up, you're probably sitting on it – what have you come for anyway?"

"I've come to see Miss Wood."

"Well why didn't you say so? I'll show you up."

As we entered her room I recalled the remark about the sun glasses. The walls were painted in bright purple gloss with an orange border!

Miss Wood lay back on her pillows and the purple gloss reflected on her face making her look at death's door. Just as I had nearly finished making her comfortable, Dr Scrimshaw came back into the room. I was looking in a drawer for a comb.

There, next to the comb, was a loose boiled sweet with hair and fluff and dandruff sticking to it.

"Ooh – look – a sweetie – shame to waste it," he cried as he pounced on it and popped it into my mouth!

* * *

The next six months were spent happily settling into the job, getting to know doctors and patients and travelling round every corner of my district. Some of the Bridgend doctors had patients on my area and even one or two patients belonged to surgeries in Hatfield or Bradford. One doctor who worked in a group practice in Bridgend had several private patients that he used to fuss over in ways his N.H.S patients never enjoyed. He would visit nearly every day and ask me to do the same. I continued to visit as necessary which resulted in regular phone calls from him along the lines of "If you could just visit every day, Mrs Ponsonby-Brown would be most grateful."Private patients were soon to become a thing of the past as these older G.P.s retired.

Meanwhile one of his private patients was Percy Cook who lived in a large house near the G.P in question. Percy had had a stroke a few years ago and Mildred his martinet of a wife needed help with his bed bath once a week.

My predecessor had been a rather large lady with hands like shovels, and at my first visit Percy looked me up and down and seemed delighted with the new model. In the bathroom, as we assembled his toilet things, Mildred was busy telling me he'd been a ladies man in his time but of course all that had stopped many years ago. She was happier with him as an invalid because at least she knew where he was.

"He can't even remember what it was about now," said Mildred, "and a good job too!"

With one of us at each side of the bed I quickly removed Percy's pyjamas and dropped a towel over his middle to preserve his modesty. As I sponged his chest I heard Mildred cry out,

"Percy! – well really!"

The towel was rising up in the middle. He obviously could remember what it was about.

* * *

Rob and I had been living in our cottage for almost two years when I started my new job. It was stone built, detached, with a date stone over the front door – 1634, and had mullioned windows. It was situated down a quiet lane in the local graveyard, as it had been a verger's cottage and it still belonged to the Church of England. Rob came to an arrangement with the vicar that in exchange for a peppercorn rent we would look after the property ourselves and we hoped to be able to buy it at some future stage.

We had no qualms about living surrounded by gravestones. The other building in the graveyard was a disused church. Built in the seventeenth century it had been abandoned in the nineteenth when one of the rich local families had built a grander church further up the road. The old church had a beautiful clock tower which was a landmark, still containing a working clock. Rob was asked to keep it wound up, which he did, until vandals broke into the building and stole the weights, silencing the old clock forever.

Our cottage could hardly be described as having all mod cons but still we loved it. The kitchen contained nothing but a sink and a few open shelves. The living room boasted a beamed ceiling and an open fire which was the only form of heating. Upstairs were two bedrooms and a tiny bathroom containing a bath and a sink.

The toilet was outside in the yard next to the coal place. It was a cold, draughty cottage, damp in places, and in winter it was not unusual to find ice on the inside of the windows. Being surrounded by fields, mice often moved in with us, finding it marginally warmer than outside. Our nearest neighbours were at a farm further down the lane. I was allowed to hang my washing out in the graveyard providing there was no funeral taking place.

* * *

"We really would be most grateful!" Mr Siddons was the Chairman of the Charity Gala Committee. To my horror he wanted me to judge the baby competition.

"I've never done anything like that before. What criteria do I use?"

"Oh – whatever you like dear; loudest scream, reddest bottom, you'll think of something ha! ha! ha!"

"How many enter?"

"Oh about a hundred usually – prolific lot round here you know! ha! ha! ha!"

"A hundred! Oh I really don't think so ..."

"Splendid my dear! I knew you wouldn't let us down"

Click – he was gone.

A letter arrived the following day confirming my agreement to judge the baby competition at the twenty fifth Annual Gala, to be held in the sports field of Lister Park. Fait accompli.

The age range was nought to eighteen months and I realized I needed to enlist two colleagues and we would split the little darlings into nought to six months, six to twelve months and twelve to eighteen months.

My friend Sue the midwife from my training days agreed to take the new babies and Edna agreed to do the middle lot after asking if she could judge the dog show instead. I would take the twelve to eighteen months.

The day of the gala dawned hot and sunny and we joined the crowd at the entrance to the field. A spotty long haired youth was directing people to their appropriate tents.

"Fancy dress third on the left," he said glancing at our uniforms.

"Don't be cheeky," I said sharply, "where's the baby competition?"

He glanced at his list. "Aha!, in the left hand corner between Save the whale and the Jesus freaks."

We found it and as we entered nearly turned round and fled. The tent was boiling hot and full of mums, dads, grannies and hot, sweating, angry babies all yelling their heads off. The spotty callow youth had been wrong about Save the whale, and we were in the next tent to the Brass Band competition, and as they tuned up the babies yelled ever louder.

A large lady with a badge on her left bosom which stated 'Administrator' bustled up to us.

"They've all got a ticket, one to er – whatever – just call them out in turn and here are your tables with weighing scales etcetera. Good luck!" and with a last glance at the mutinous babies, she fled.

As I took my seat a family on the front row of my lot was waving at me vigorously.

"Hello Sister! We've brought Humphrey!"

I ministered to the Grundys and all their children on a regular basis with head lice, scabies, impetigo and most other complaints in the unsavoury category.

Due to a recent influx of Disciples of Jesus Christ of the Latter Day Saints in the area, they had recently become Mormons. Most often these young men were lucky to get a foot over the threshold, but since no one in the Grundy household worked, they were received with open arms as light relief from their usual occupation of watching old American films on television and a pleasant change from debt collectors or the bailiffs.

Having become Mormons they had had their last four children baptized as a job lot at the church of their new faith, amid much rejoicing by the Mormons who'd been having a bit of a thin time of it convert wise. Strongly influenced by the old American films and probably thinking it would please the Mormons, their last two babies were named Mickey Rooney Grundy and Humphrey Bogart Grundy.

Mother, father and an obese Humphrey Bogart Grundy sat in front of me whilst I asked about his diet.

"He can down a plate of fish and chips faster than the dog," Dad claimed proudly.

"Can I see your teeth Humphrey?" I asked, putting my hand on his chin.

He beamed and spat a large sticky toffee into my palm. Mrs Grundy seized it and dropped it on to the grass.

"Eeeh lad! – you don't know where nurses' hands have been."

The afternoon wore on relentlessly with baby following baby, the tent getting hotter and the bands next door hardly pausing for breath, until like a prize cabbage a winner of each category was chosen, followed by an overall winner. The photographer from the local paper took his pictures and sensing a somewhat surly atmosphere, and realising we had made enemies of all the non winners, we slunk out of the back of the tent muttering 'never again'.

* * *

Ethel Brown was fast becoming my *bête noir.* An old lady in her eighties she lived alone in a small cottage. It was vital for old people to keep mobile – to move around in their homes and if possible outside, or they simply seized up altogether and their legs would no longer support them. The Geriatric Consultant saw many patients like this when doing domiciliary visits and he would simply call it "gone off his/her legs." He would then have to take them into hospital for a short time, mainly for physiotherapy to get them weight bearing and mobile again.

Ethel had more or less decided she didn't want to bother walking about any more. She would just stay on the settee in front of the fire with her radio and television. Her nice neighbour would do her shopping, she would have a home help to keep the house clean and tidy, meals on wheels would bring her a hot meal every other day and the nice district nurse would wash and change her and see to her toileting needs.

And so we started going round in circles. Ethel would become so stiff and immobile that I couldn't budge her from the settee. Her legs would swell up and she would become incontinent. I would ask the G.P to arrange for the Geriatrician to visit and the ambulance service to carry Ethel up to bed. Then I would have to visit at least twice daily, locking her in at night while we waited for a hospital bed to become available. She would go to hospital where after a week or two of intensive physiotherapy from the staff she would come home again, where she sat on her couch and quickly deteriorated and started the whole thing off again.

I communicated with the hospital consultant through the Geriatric Liaison Officer – a qualified district nurse, who as far as Ethel Brown was concerned quickly became piggy in the middle between me and the consultant. Tony was a very gentle and polite young man. The phone would ring and there he was, telling me Ethel was coming home again – and I would hit the roof. Eventually Tony became so terrified of my reaction he would talk about other patients and at the end say – "if I could just whisper E.B?"

Well, here she was coming home again. I settled her in and told her she must go up the stairs to bed at night and keep herself mobile.

"Of course I'll go upstairs, don't natter me!"

"Well you don't usually do you?"

"Aye well 'appen I've mended me ways. I don't want to go back in hospital."

Ethel had mended her ways! This I had to see. It lasted a week before she took to her usual spot on the settee. Then I had to start evening visits to man-handle her up the narrow stone stairs and into bed, where she would tuck all sorts of cardigans and towels round herself 'in case'. There was no 'in case' about it, every morning she would be wet through as she had no hope of getting to the bathroom unaided.

"You'll have to go back into hospital Ethel; you can't stay on your own like this."

"I'm not going."

"Ethel, how do you think I feel – locking you in at night and leaving you helpless?"

"I know – how can you fashion?" There was no answer to that.

A week later I finally got Ethel back into hospital and this time she didn't come home again. Do you know I rather missed her.

* * *

When I first visited Mary and George they were trying to come to terms with the fact that she was dying of breast cancer.

"If I can just know that I can stay at home I can cope," Mary said.

47

She told me and the G.P that she had had enough of hospitals. We promised her she could be cared for at home and this seemed to put her mind at rest.

Mary had been a librarian but for many years had helped George run his health food shop. They were also vegetarians but the vegetable regime combined with the health foods seemed to have done them very little good as they were both pale and pasty and one of the most unhealthy couples I'd ever met. Mary had been in and out of hospital for years having first one breast off and then the other plus chemotherapy and radiotherapy.

Now her time was limited. She was in a most pathetic condition with her chest wall eroded and bleeding and her arms heavy with fluid, having had her lymph nodes removed. She was unable to move her arms at all and the journey to the bathroom for daily washing before I attended to her dressings became gradually more difficult. However, it was a pleasure to visit her as she always remained cheerful and courageous. We would find plenty to chat about and George would be ready with a cup of tea when I came downstairs again.

One thing which was quite worrying was the possibility that a haemorrhage would occur from the eroded chest wall so I had adrenaline ready for emergencies on the dressing tray.

The weeks passed by but Mary was getting weaker. One night my phone rang at three a.m. George's anxious voice roused me from sleep.

"Mary started bleeding heavily about half an hour ago and she collapsed on the floor so I rang for the doctor and a different one came."

"Do you want me as well George?" I asked, reluctant to get out of my warm bed.

"Well he's gone and Mary's still on the floor – I can't move her and she's semi conscious."

This didn't make sense. "Hang on George – I'm on my way"

I jumped quickly into uniform and set off into the February night. When I arrived it was just as George said. Mary was on the bedroom floor too weak to move or speak, but at least the bleeding had stopped.

"What did the doctor do?" I asked.

"Nothing – he took a quick look at Mary and said she must go into hospital. Mary managed to say she didn't want to go, she wanted to die at home and he said 'you are causing your own suffering' and then he went out to the car. I thought he'd gone to fetch something but he just drove off, so I rang you."

I managed to push the rage I felt at this to the back of my mind and concentrate on Mary and their plight. An hour later when she was clean and comfortable in bed and drowsy from her oral morphia, she whispered "thank you."

The following morning Mary's visit was an early priority. She was very weak.

"The moment I saw your black stockings and shoes come round the door I knew I'd be alright," she managed to whisper. It is still one of the nicest things anyone has ever said to me. A few days later Mary died peacefully in her bed at home.

Chapter 4

Work wise I was just beginning to feel more confident and getting into my stride when I discovered I was pregnant. I had only been in my new post for six months and remembering Miss Burton's question at my interview about working mothers, I had mixed feelings about the situation, although, work apart, Rob and I were delighted.

"Don't you think it is a baby's birthright to be cared for by it's mother at home Mrs Baines?" Miss Burton asked sternly.

I had arranged for my overjoyed mother-in-law, who lived only half a mile away, to care for the baby during working hours, but this cut no ice with Miss Burton. Under recent legislation paid maternity leave was eleven weeks before the birth and seven after and woe betide you if baby was late and you took twelve weeks before as I did.

"Do you think it's fair to your colleagues to be off for so long Sister?"

I was to be the first nurse under her charge to take this maternity leave and she was so disapproving, from that moment on I was to be forever in her bad books – not however a difficult place to get to.

I staggered somehow through the first three months of my pregnancy feeling and being terribly sick and not daring to take leave. Just as the nausea was diminishing and I was coping better I grew more like humpty-dumpty by the day until I was waddling round covering my bump with my apron and trying to keep out of sight of Miss B. I was more than relieved to reach my twenty-ninth week as the steering wheel was scraping on my bump.

Our baby daughter arrived safely, the summer getting to know each other flew by and before I knew it I was back on duty. My new routine was quite exhausting. Up early, feed and change baby, drop baby at Gran's, do a hefty mornings work, back to Grans for a quick lunch and feed and change baby again, work again then pick up baby and home to cook evening meal and hope there were no evening visits. Lucy was a good baby but naturally she had to be fed during the night and as I was feeding her myself no-one else could help.

The hardest thing was the cold of the first winter. We had fitted a night storage heater in the baby's room but the house was still bitterly cold. There was no time to light a fire in the morning so we used fan heaters in the living room and the kitchen. I sometimes wondered how I survived that first year, and I take my hat off to all the previous generations of selfless women who've fed babies in the night in freezing cold rooms.

My patients were all glad to see me back and wanted to hear about Lucy and her progress. Edna had had to have help from the Bridgend nurses during my maternity leave and was also relieved that I was back on duty.

Shortly after my return the phone rang at about seven in the evening. It was Dr Galbraith senior asking me to visit old Mr Craddock just up the road, who was suffering from a bad case of constipation.

"Och! – I wouldn't bother you lassie were it not for his women folk – they're making such a fuss!"

I was met at the door of the Craddock household by two elderly ladies; his wife and her sister. Mr Craddock and his wife were almost stone deaf and more than a bit senile. Fortunately her sister had come to live with them and she was a sensible old lady.

"Oh come in – come in," they chorused together, delighted to see me.

Mr Craddock was sitting in his armchair seemingly unconcerned. The ladies stood wringing their hands with the horror of it all.

"You see, my dear," said the sister, dropping her voice to a stage whisper aimed at my right ear, "he hasn't been!"

My patient grinned and nodded when I introduced myself and I asked the ladies to help him up to bed whilst I prepared my equipment in the kitchen. The disposable enema was years in the future and it was still our habit to attack our patients with pints of hot soapy water pumped through yards of rubber tubing. In fact little had changed since the days of Florence Nightingale and our triumph in the Crimea may have owed something to the fact that men preferred to stay and fight rather than report sick and be given an enema.

Preparations complete, I carried my tray of weaponry to the stairs to discover Mr Craddock, bent double with arthritis, but grinning and nodding, had just about reached the top step. Helping him on to his bed I explained what I was about to do.

I asked if he would co-operate by retaining the fluid, preferably until I got him into the bathroom, and realised by the now familiar grin and nod that he hadn't the vaguest idea what I was talking about. My spirits sank as I knew that as fast as I pumped the fluid in, not only would he not retain it, but would probably blow it back at me. The bed would be soaked, I would be soaked, Mr Craddock would still be constipated and the ladies would be left ringing their hands.

I placed my patient in the left lateral position and began. Slowly the level of fluid in the jug went down and amazingly disappeared from sight. The bed remained dry! Mr Craddock seemed not to have noticed anything had happened. I had surely done him an injustice! He was the perfect patient.

I helped him from the bed and as we headed towards the bathroom I realised why things had gone well so far. The curvature of his spine was trapping the liquid in his bowel. When he was comfortably settled, I joined the ladies to boil my equipment and put it away in my bag. Confident of a successful result I told them not to worry, everything was under control.

I returned to Mr Craddock and helped him rise from the toilet seat and looked into the bowl expecting to see the answer to all our problems – nothing! I sat him down again and exhorted him to greater effort – nothing! My training had not prepared me for this eventuality. If Sister Tutor had known it was possible to lose, without trace, two pints of fluid inside a patient, she had kept it a very dark secret. Deciding to have another look I helped Mr Craddock to get up again. His joints were by this time so stiff that instead of rising, his head bent forward to touch the floor and his bottom rose in the air.

As his spine straightened there was a loud explosion and two pints of soapy water plus the contents of Mr Craddock's bowel made a desperate bid for freedom.

The evil smelling brown liquid flew upwards and fanned out in an ever increasing spiral as I stood, too shocked to move. When it stopped, the walls had changed colour; the ceiling had changed colour; I had changed colour. The only place that had not changed colour was the toilet; it twinkled and gleamed up at me in hygienic mockery.

"Well?" asked Mr Craddock. Neither of us had yet moved a muscle. We still stood side by side, nurse holding patient.

"Well what?" I managed to say in flat tones.

"Have I been?"

"Oh – yes, you've been!" What more was there to say?

I helped him back to his room after a quick wash and brush up. The ladies met me in the hall with hope shining from their faces.

"Has he been?" they chorused together.

"Well yes he's been, but I'm afraid the bathroom's a bit of a mess."

"Oh that's alright dear. We're so grateful to you, don't worry about a little thing like that!" said the sensible one.

It was funny they didn't seem to notice that my uniform was no longer the fresh clean one I had arrived in and that my aura was anything but fragrant. How could I tell them that the bathroom needed fumigating and redecorating.

"But I must explain......"

"Nonsense dear, we'll tidy up. Now off you go and enjoy the rest of your evening!" – and I left them waving and calling words of everlasting gratitude from the doorstep.

* * *

We were starting to improve the cottage by putting a toilet in to the bathroom. No more creeping out into the yard in all weathers to an outside loo which invariably froze up in winter. Heaven!

The next job was the kitchen. The floor was stone flags and there had been a fireplace in one corner which was sealed off.

"If I take this wall down it will give us more space," Rob said as he hit the wall with a huge stone hammer. We cleared away the rubble and Rob started to sweep the floor where the grate had been.

"There's some writing on this flagstone." he said, sweeping away the soot and dust.

"What does it say?" I asked with curiosity.

"Here lies – the body – of – John – son of William," Rob said slowly.

I screamed "Oh – there's a body under our kitchen floor!"

Rob soon decided that when they had rebuilt the cottage in 1866, moving it from the top end of the graveyard next to the church, as stated on a plaque on the back wall, they had used a gravestone as a hearthstone. He assured me that John, son of William, was not buried in our kitchen.

There were to be further repercussions of living in close proximity to the deceased when Lucy started school. Her nursery teacher asked to speak to me to voice her concerns about Lucy's art work.

"I'm quite worried Mrs Baines, all the pictures she draws or paints are full of crosses and tombstones!"

I re-assured her that Lucy had a graveyard for a garden and thought nothing of it. Her first composition was entitled "The view from my bedroom window."

Lucy wrote:- 'From my bedroom window I can see Walter Greenwood's grave'.

There were quite a few children at school who had beautiful gardens with swings and slides but 'Lucy's house' was always the favourite venue to be invited to tea because of playing in the graveyard.

* * *

It was late afternoon and the light was fading as I was finishing my last patient on a new housing estate which was still being built. Dropping my bag onto the back seat I felt a tugging at my coat.

"Please, please, you've got to come – my wife is having a baby!" An agitated man of about thirty-five was trying to pull me across the road to his house.

"Hang on a minute – I'm not a midwife. Have you sent for an ambulance, or a midwife?"

"Yes! Yes! but the baby's coming now! now! oh please come!"

I felt I had no choice and that I couldn't just get in the car and drive off. I followed him through the gloom and into a brightly lit and beautifully decorated hallway. My new patient was standing at the bottom of the stairs, yelling her head off.

I told them my name and found out they were Joanne and Malcolm, and it was their second child and they had only moved in the previous week. Not enjoying being in hospital with her first delivery, Joanne had decided to hang on as long as she could and had obviously left it too late.

A cursory examination told me the baby's head was on the perineum and I had to get Joanne lying down.

"I'm not lying down here! This carpet is brand new and cost a fortune!" Her fingers tightened on the banisters.

Malcolm was running up and down like a headless chicken. I grabbed him as he ran past.

"Malcolm! Go and fetch me lots of clean towels or sheets – then ring the ambulance service again."

"Yes, yes! towels! sheets! – ambulance!" he repeated it like a mantra as he took the stairs two at a time. Joanne was not so easily biddable.

"Let's get you into the living room and on to the couch Joanne," I said firmly, trying to prise her fingers off the banister.

"I'm not going on the couch – it's brand new – it cost a fortune!" she yelled glaring at me.

It was time to take charge of the situation.

"Well you can't stay here, the baby is ready to be born," I said firmly, "stop being a silly girl!"

Malcolm appeared with enough sheets and towels to start a market stall and as I heaved Joanne into the living room we heard him say, "I've rung before – please hurry – we're having a baby!"

"What's this '**we**' Malcolm?" Joanne yelled, "I'm having a baby, not you Malcolm – you blockhead!" As I lowered Joanne on to a well protected couch, Malcolm called in panic. "She wants to know where we live – where do we live?"

"Four Beechwood Road! – Malcolm – you blockhead!" It was quite common for mums to be aggressive at this stage of labour and Joanne was directing it all at the hapless Malcolm.

I instructed Joanne to pant and not to push as Malcolm rushed in with the news that the ambulance would be here any minute. We felt a breeze on our faces; Malcolm was puffing and panting along with Joanne.

"Not you Malcolm – you don't need to pant – blockhead!" came Joanne's predictable cry.

Just as the baby's head was appearing a paramedic walked in and I'd never been so glad to see one. Pulling sterile gloves on, he delivered the baby as I slipped out of the room to leave them to it. I heard the baby's first cries and Malcolm's voice.

"Ohh look! – it's a baby – a lovely little baby!"

I could hear Joanne's reply as I climbed gratefully into my car.

"Of course it's a baby Malcolm – what were you expecting – a three toed sloth? – Blockhead!"

* * *

"Ah! Sister Baines!" Miss Burton pounced on me as I called in at the Health Department for some equipment. I groaned silently as it was after lunch time and I was starving.

"Dr Carter rang with a visit for Sister Stubs but she's gone home feeling ill, so you can do it – it's an Asian gentleman on Balaclava Terrace for an enema. Dr Carter says he doesn't envy you as he speaks very little English." She looked very pleased with herself as she passed me the message.

Half an hour later I was at four Balaclava Terrace. My efforts to be understood started in the kitchen with four silent ladies of varying ages. Three brown toddlers were chasing a hen round the yard.

"Hello – I'm Sister Baines. Where is Mr Ahmed?" brought blank stares.

Hearing men's voices in the front room I thought I would try there instead. At first the question got the same blank stares from the five men in there, until one said "Mr Ahmed" and pointed at the ceiling.

I made my way up the stairs. I would come down again to fight for a jug of hot water and towels after I had explained to the patient. Mr Ahmed, a young man of about thirty-five was in the back bedroom holding his stomach and groaning loudly. His big brown eyes watched me warily as I opened my bag and pulled out my Higginson's syringe and rectal catheter and placed them on a small table at the side of the bed.

I explained to him that Dr Carter had asked me to give him an enema and realised, with a sinking heart, that he hadn't understood a word. I decided to mime the procedure. Holding the apparatus, I mimed – "I – am – going – to put this – up there – and scoot– two pints – of hot – soapy water – through this – tube – into – your rectum."

His eyes grew large with horror and he clutched the sheet to his chin. Finally he let out a roar.

"You – mad – English – woman!!!" and suddenly he leapt out of bed and stampeded to the toilet at the end of the corridor. Judging by the noises that emanated from the room, my visit had been a great success without laying a finger on him. As I left, the men downstairs greeted me with smiles and nods and even a small round of applause.

* * *

Miss Amelia Hudd-Smith was a refined and cultured old lady of ninety-two, who refused to let the modern world intrude upon her. Imperious and Victorian, she was always in command of the situation, just as she had been as headmistress of a girls' school, thirty-five years before.

She shared a house with her friend and companion, Miss Brook, at eighty-seven the younger of the two. Miss Brook had also been a teacher in her working days. Although one might describe them as being in reduced circumstances, they had both come from 'good families', and consequently could afford a daily help to do the shopping and keep the house clean, and a gardener for a few hours a week. They kept very much to themselves, and were able to remain independent – until Miss Hudd-Smith overbalanced in the garden one afternoon and broke her arm.

For the first time in her life she was taken by ambulance to hospital where, following an x-ray, her hand and arm were immobilised in a plaster of Paris cast. Being rather shocked, and in any case having no choice, she co-operated with dignity and quietly determined she would never go there again.

I called to see her the following day in case she needed any help with toileting. She had managed, however, with the help of the faithful Miss Brook – a much less robust old lady, who looked as if she could do with some help herself due to arthritis of the spine.

"Never mind, six weeks will soon pass and then you'll be able to have your pot off." I smiled at Miss Hudd-Smith.

"Will Dr Galbraith take it off?" she enquired. Dr Galbraith senior was her G.P. and an old friend.

"No. I'm afraid you'll have to go back to the hospital – you have an appointment in six weeks time."

"Oh – no dear!" she smiled sweetly at me, "I shall not go there again, I didn't like it at all."

I opened my mouth to tell her that of course she would have to go, when I caught sight of Miss Brook standing behind her, shaking her head.

"Better leave it for now dear, we don't want to upset her," she said at the door, "thank you for calling."

Six weeks passed and I had quite forgotten about Miss Hudd-Smith and her pot, when Dr Galbraith asked me to call again.

"Can you see if you can get the plaster off? – she refuses to go back to the fracture clinic"

"I can't get that off, Doctor – it needs a plaster saw! She'll have to go to hospital."

"Well, I canny persuade her – when she says no, she means it. See if you can work it loose a wee bit – it's bound to have softened round the edges – or maybe you could soak it off?" he said hopefully.

I looked unconvinced. He put his arm on mine persuasively. "Have a wee try lassie – just for me."

At the cottage Miss Brook told me how the ambulance men had called twice for Miss Hudd-Smith, and she had behaved as graciously as the Queen Mother at a garden party, but refused to go.

"How nice of you to call," she had told them, "but my arm feels very comfortable and I really don't need to have the plaster off. I've quite got used to it now. Thank you for coming to see me – goodbye!" and she had shut the door firmly in their faces.

Dr Galbraith had called three times but she remained impervious to his attempts at persuasion, un-impressed by his arguments. It seemed I was the last hope. Unless I could persuade her where others had failed, she would carry the pot to her grave.

A swift examination at least ruled out any attempt to take it off at home. It was far too thick to soak off and it had not softened round the edges – it was in fact a credit to the plaster room attendant who had applied it.

"Now wouldn't it be a relief to get it off, Miss Hudd-Smith? It must be so hot and heavy."

"No, not at all – I like it – and I didn't like that hospital. Now please don't fuss – you're as bad as Dr Galbraith!" – and she laid her head back and closed her eyes. I had been dismissed.

Miss Brook escorted me off the premises. At the door I had an idea, born of desperation.

"Do you think she would go if I took her in my car, instead of the ambulance?" Miss Brook looked doubtful.

"Tell her we could drive past her school on the way." I knew Miss Hudd-Smith had maintained her interest in the school and loved to see the girls in their uniform coming and going.

"Well," said Miss Brook slowly, "I can ask her – it may work – we haven't been to the school for some time."

"Tell her I've promised Dr Galbraith I'll get the plaster off and I'm quite worried about it. Tell her anything, but we must get it off!" Surprisingly, Miss Hudd-Smith relented.

"Oh, very well – if only to stop you all going on about it, but I shan't stay long at the hospital, I really didn't like it." I telephoned the fracture clinic and spoke to my colleague in charge.

"I'm bringing her at 2 o'clock on Thursday – for heaven's sake get her straight in to see the doctor and have the plaster room technician standing by, before she changes her mind. I'll never be able to get her back again so it's a now or never job!"

"Right – let me know the minute you arrive and you can be next in."

On the Thursday I arrived to collect the old ladies, more than half expecting Miss Hudd-Smith to have changed her mind. They were both ready with hats and coats on. Miss Brook looked agitated.

"It's one of her bad days, she can't remember anything from one minute to the next. She can't remember having promised to go to the hospital."

"Where are we going?" Miss Hudd-Smith demanded, glaring at me.

"We're going for a drive to see the school," I lied, or half lied. I installed them in the back seat of the car. Miss Hudd-Smith sat regally in silence. About a mile from the hospital an indignant voice sailed from the back into my left ear.

"I think it's disgraceful!" she announced – to no-one in particular. "One is sitting quietly at home, minding one's own business, when one is bundled into a motorcar and driven 'orf, without the slightest idea where one is going!"

That was all, she didn't speak another word. At the hospital I positively hustled them into the out-patients hall. I found them seats next to the consulting room door and dashed off to let my colleague know we had arrived.

"Right! I'll get you in next, – she can see Dr. Grieve, the registrar."

I returned to sit with my charges, praying we wouldn't have long to wait. The out-patients hall was crowded as usual. About thirty people sat waiting their turn to see a doctor, have a plaster removed, or have an x-ray. Old men coughed and wheezed, bored children dragged on and off their mother's knees. Miss Hudd-Smith sat erect, clutching her handbag on her knee, surveying her fellow beings in utter disgust. Being slightly deaf, her voice rang out probably much louder than she intended.

"Who are all these dreadful people?"

The comment echoed round the waiting room, silencing all other conversation. All eyes turned towards us. I felt like crawling beneath my chair, but Miss Hudd-Smith stared back, quite unrepentant.

"'Ere – 'oo d'ya think you're calling dreadful?" demanded a fat aggressive looking woman, indignantly. The situation looked like becoming nasty, when suddenly the door behind us opened and Miss Hudd-Smith's name was called. I rushed her in with relief, leaving poor Miss Brook to sit it out with the dreadful people.

The registrar looked irritable and overworked. Quickly I explained to him that the plaster had been in position for twelve weeks instead of the customary six. He looked at the x-rays.

"Lets have it removed then – it was a fairly simple fracture. I'll have a look at her wrist when the pot's off to see if she should come for some physiotherapy." He addressed me, ignoring Miss Hudd-Smith completely. She had no intention of tolerating such rude behaviour.

"Young man," she glared at him, her imperious tone demanding his attention. "Kindly do not discuss me as if I were not here!" And raising her plastered arm she caught him a neat blow in the middle of his bald forehead. I frog-marched her out before he could recover himself. In the plaster room, the attendant eyed her warily.

An electric saw is a frightening appliance and it wouldn't have been surprising if she had decided to make a fight of it, but, made of the stuff that had once ruled an empire, Miss Hudd-Smith sat with quiet dignity until the cast lay on the plaster room floor.

Relief almost overwhelmed me when I had delivered them back to their home. I telephoned Dr Galbraith from the clinic to let him share in the good news.

"Och! I knew you'd do it lassie" he was delighted. "Well done! Well done! You deserve the Victoria Cross, and I'll see that you get it!"

I'm still waiting ......

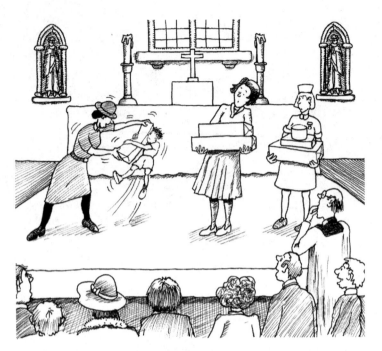

Chapter 5

The vicar of one of the local churches seemed to have taken a shine to me. I came to his notice as I was visiting his mother-in-law who lived in a bed-sit at the manse. Celia was in her nineties and was one of my favourites. She came from a county family, was very well spoken and had led a fascinating life. She had been a V.A.D nurse in France during World War I, had driven an ambulance in London in the Blitz in her sixties in World War II, and she and her late husband had counted Winston and Clementine Churchill, and the composer Delius as friends.

I looked forward to my weekly visit to Celia, she was so interesting to talk to, but the vicar would always pounce on me with some request or other.

"I wonder if you could come and give our cubs and scouts some lectures on first aid?"

"Er – some? I don't mind doing one."

"Oh splendid! And perhaps a mother-craft class for our girl scouts? Well done!"

His head disappeared round the door before I could protest.

"Bloody cheek!" Celia had heard all. "You should have told him to push off!"

As a committed atheist, Celia could not get over the fact that she had ended up living with a son-in-law who was a man of the cloth, in a vicarage. Although she never missed a chance to pour scorn on his head, often in delightfully ripe language, it was my opinion she was secretly very fond of him and grateful that she had been given a loving and comfortable home with her daughter.

As it was nearly Christmas his latest idea was a present giving service, when the parishioners would donate a gift for a sick or deprived child, to be attended by the matron of a children's home, a nurse from the children's ward of the local hospital, and me. I explained this to Celia during the coffee and chat we always had after her injection; at least I had coffee whilst Celia had a tot of whisky and a cigarette in a long cigarette holder. She muttered darkly about not trusting 'that lot' to cough up anything worth having.

"Geoffrey dragged me along to the Mother's Union once – of course they all think Geoffrey is wonderful. A strange little woman in a hand knitted fair-isle cardigan, with a pudding basin hair cut, asked me how many children I had and didn't I think having them was the greatest achievement of my life? I said she hadn't met my children and two of them should have been drowned at birth and I could think of far better things I'd done with my life!"

Lucy was three years old now and Rob and I explained that she had to choose a toy to give the 'poor children' at the service. She was all for it as it meant a trip to her favourite shop and a good rummage through the latest delights. She chose a fire engine and we duly wrapped it in Christmassy paper and labelled it suitable for a boy aged three to five years.

The day dawned and we sat in church near the front. Towards the end of the service the vicar announced the giving of presents.

"With out hearts full of Jesus' love for those less fortunate than ourselves, and to be received by our guests, Matron from the children's home, a nurse from the children's ward, and – his voice rising – **our very own district nurse!"** I half expected the organ to go –da-da-da-da-da-dah!

We stood on the platform at the front of the church as the worshippers and young children came up with their wrapped offerings. Lucy came up with her chosen present and gave it to me looking a bit miffed about something.

"Where are the poor children, Mummy?" she asked in a very loud voice, "I want to see them!"

The next little boy held out his gift half heartedly and as I took it he changed his mind.

"Let go pet," I said tugging in vain.

"But I like it, its mine!" he wailed, his lip trembling.

"No it's not, let go," I muttered through my teeth, finally winning the undignified battle as he ran back to his mother howling. I made a mental note not to come to this service ever again.

It made a good story to tell Celia. Unfortunately a lot of the presents turned out to be anything but new and many not fit to give to a child. Celia snorted scornfully. "What did I tell you? Miserable stingy lot of buggers!"

* * *

"I've had some good news this morning, I can't wait to tell you about it."

Mrs Gregory was another of my favourites. It was Wednesday morning and I was helping her to have a shower. She suffered from rheumatoid arthritis, making all her joints stiff and painful, but as usual she had a smile on her face and she tried not to complain.

"Come on then what's new?" I asked as I turned the shower on to a gentle spray.

"Do you remember when I told you about that lovely lady who came to see me from the British Legion?"

"Oh yes – they helped you buy a new cooker didn't they?"

"Well she's written to ask if I'd like to go to one of their holiday homes for a week – its at Southport, and if I'd find it difficult on my own I can take a carer so I'm going to ask my cousin Betty. She can't afford a holiday either. Isn't it wonderful?"

"Lovely – just what you need. Send me a postcard!"

Mrs Gregory had had a hard life. She had no children and had lost her husband in the Second World War. He had been the love of her life and photo's of him in his

R.A.F uniform were all over the house. She had never married again.

"Oh no dear – I'd never find anyone like my Alf – although I had my chances!" she would tell me with a twinkle in her eye. She was very hard up trying to manage on her pensions, her war widows' pension taking her just above the level where she could claim benefits. Living in her own home didn't help. There was no spare money for repairs or replacements.

"Mrs Haley – that's the lady from the British Legion – asked me if I'd ever had any help from them before and I asked her if 1922 counted as it's nearly fifty years ago."

I was drying her now, noticing how frail she looked and how her knees creaked audibly as they took her weight.

"You must have been quite young then, just after the First World War?" I was interested to hear about it.

"I was eight and the eldest of five children."

"Well, go on – tell me about it!"

Mrs Gregory laughed, "That's what she said!"

We were downstairs now and just about to have a cuppa. Mrs Gregory settled into her special chair with relief.

"Well, after the First World War, the men who were lucky enough to come back weren't the same men who'd gone away. My father came home in 1919 but his nerves were bad. He suffered from terrible depression. He'd sit in sullen silence most of the time, shouting at us kids if we made a noise. I don't know how my mother coped with him at all especially as he worked at home. He had a shed in the garden where he mended shoes – he couldn't get anything better – a land fit for heroes and no jobs for them. Then he started hitting Mother when he lost his temper. He used to fly into rages all the time – we were all terrified of him but I don't think he could help it. One day he hit Mother and her lip was cut and her face was all bruised. She'd just had a baby and wasn't very strong. She was trying to feed the baby but I don't think she had enough milk as we never had enough food, and we were both crying.

Dad had gone out to the shed and Mother made some tea and told me to fetch him. I was frightened of disturbing him and stood outside for ages. Then I opened the door."

She was silent and I noticed her hand shaking, holding her tea-cup.

"I'll never forget what I saw. He was lying back on some sacks; there was blood in pools on the floor – he'd cut his throat. I dreamt about what I saw for years. Mother collapsed in shock and I had to run and fetch a neighbour. The police came and Mother was taken to hospital with the baby and I was left to look after my sister and two little brothers. We'd no money and no food. Some neighbours brought bits of food round but no-one could spare much. One lady gave me a dish of crusts they'd cut off their bread – literally sparing a crust! There were no social services then you know. Then some-one told the British Legion about us. They came and brought us food and gave us money and kept an eye on us until Mother came home."

As I left Mrs Gregory, clean and comfortable again, I marvelled at the spirit that had kept her going, cheerful and positive through all the adversity in her life.

* * *

I was having a somewhat trying morning. Visiting a remote house at the edge of my district, almost on moor land, my patient was being very slow to answer the door, which was locked. I called through the letterbox and finally an old lady in a dressing gown appeared in the hallway. She fiddled with bars and bolts on the door for what seemed like ages and then said. "Oh! I've got the wrong key," and disappeared again.

I looked at my watch impatiently – I'd been here ten minutes already and I hadn't even got in yet. She appeared again and called to me, "I can't find the key. Go round the back and I'll open the patio door." I made my way round the back, snagging a new pair of black tights on a prickly bush. Reaching the patio door I could see Mrs Smith walking slowly towards the door when – disaster! – she tripped over a rug and fell heavily on to her side, catching her head on a coffee table. My patient was lying injured and bleeding, probably with a fractured femur, and I was locked out unable to help!

I had no choice but to tell her I was going for help and would be back soon and I drove off to the first house I came to about three quarters of a mile away. Soon, police and ambulance were on their way following me down the lane. They were able to break in and shortly Mrs Smith was in the ambulance and I could leave telling the relatives to the police. I had wasted an hour of my day.

A new patient was next, back in the village, and I arrived at the door of his rather grand house, opposite the golf course, just as Dr Galbraith junior was coming out.

"He can't wait to meet you," he said, and burst out laughing. On the door was pinned a note which said. Do come straight in Nursie. I can't wait to meet you!

My G.P's always found the situation hilarious when I had lecherous old men to deal with.

Mr Gardener had a reputation as an old roué who had led his wife, lady captain at the golf club, a merry dance until she left him. I sent up a silent prayer that the dressing I had to change wouldn't be anywhere near his private parts. He was wearing pyjamas and a dressing gown as we made our way into the bedroom. I got my sterile dressing pack ready and discreetly folded his pyjamas away from the wound area on his lower abdomen, and turned to the sink to wash my hands. Turning back I let out a squeal of shock to find him stark naked on the bed.

"What's wrong my dear? You've seen a naked man before haven't you?"

I mentally kicked myself for showing a reaction. Po-faced and without saying a word I changed the dressing as he rambled on about where he would take me to dinner when he was allowed out.

"I'll see you again tomorrow Mr Gardener." I said, picking up my bag to leave.

"I'm looking forward to it and I shall be undressed ready for you Nursie," he leered.

"You really should cover yourself up," and glancing at his middle portion, "it's cold – you've nearly disappeared!" I said, hoping a put down would cure him.

Calling round to see Celia for a coffee break, I told her about my encounter with the geriatric Casanova. She realised who I meant straight away.

"The silly old bugger!" she exclaimed. "You should take out a big knife and chop his plums 'orf!"

* * *

Hubert Wainwright was another ladies man. A large ungainly chap, he'd led his wife a miserable life with one infidelity after another. No one could understand why she had put up with him and perhaps she had planned to leave after the children had grown up and flown the nest. If she had, sadly, she'd left it too late as she became seriously ill and I nursed her at home for a few weeks before she died.

Hubert didn't seem too upset during her illness and following an evening visit he met me at the bottom of the stairs with a large sherry, despite my protests, and an invitation to join him for a drink. If I had assumed this was his attempt at seduction however, I couldn't have been more wrong.

"I'm just writing some poetry to try to impress my lady love, she's rather well read you know, loves literature and poetry."

Considering his wife was lying on her death bed upstairs, my face must have been a picture of shock and disapproval.

"Oh – Marion and I have been daggers drawn for years – should've split up long ago. She wouldn't thank me for pretending otherwise now. I'll give her a good send off – it's all I can do."

I was stunned by his frankness and prepared to either drink the sherry, or pour it onto the nearest pot plant and leave. Just then the phone rang and Hubert hurried off into the hall and I found I couldn't resist a peek at his poetic efforts to impress his 'well read' lady friend:-

I love you in your dressing gown.
I love you in your nightie,
but when the moonlight flits
Across your tits.

Jesus Christ Almighty!

Hmmm – that should do it Hubert.

* * *

As I pulled into the car park of the health department I noticed a small bright purple car with a large sun flower painted on the side. Sitting outside the nurses' office was the owner – my new student for the next two weeks.

Susie, Nurse Carlson, was almost as colourful as her car.

She was dressed in a green jacket over a very short pink mini skirt. Someone in authority had had the bright idea of allowing student nurses to go out on the district wearing mufti. The sight of her was enough to give some of my elderly gentlemen a heart attack.

Most students were shy or nervous on their first day out in the community with an unknown sister and I usually spent time trying to put them at their ease. Not necessary with Susie; she was an extrovert and before we reached the first patient I learned what my reputation among the current student nurses was.

"So I said to Nurse Wilson – she's the student you had two months ago – I'm going to Newholme with Sister Baines, what's she like? and Nurse Wilson said "Oh she's okay as long as you don't smoke or eat garlic!"

I marvelled at the extent of the good points in my favour, as I pulled up at the first house.

"This patient is suffering from rheumatoid arthritis and her mobility is very poor. She has also had an abdoperineal resection of rectum and she needs help to care for her colostomy until she gets used to it and gains confidence. Have you nursed a patient like this before Nurse Carlson?"

"Oh yes, loads," said Nurse Carlson stepping out onto the pavement showing an alarming amount of leg and other bodily parts.

"Oh good." I said, "perhaps you'll be able to write an account of the required nursing care for your homework at the end of the week."

Our next patient had pernicious anemia and of course Nurse Carlson knew all about that as well. I asked if she could explain the intrinsic factor.

"Ah well," she began hesitantly, but a dog shot across the front of the car causing me to brake suddenly and by the time we had collected ourselves the moment had passed.

I was rather looking forward to the next visit which was to Mr Gardener my old roué, to see what he would make of Nurse Carlson and her mini skirt.

He was waiting in the bedroom, scantily dressed as usual. I introduced them, watching Mr Gardener's eyes popping out of his head.

"If you wash your hands Nurse you can prepare Mr Gardener and take his dressing off." I busied myself preparing the sterile dressing pack.

"What a lovely young lady you are! How lucky I am to have two beautiful ladies to care for me," babbled Mr Gardener, lying back on his bed and gazing from one to the other of us. His hand wandered over the edge of the bed and he tentatively ran it up Susie's leg. She squealed and slapped it away. It was lovely not to be on the receiving end for once.

"I'm very pleased with the wound now," I told him, "just keep this dressing on for another day and then it will be healed perfectly – no need for any further visits – ready Nurse Carlson?" I headed for the door.

"But Nursie! We haven't talked about when I'm taking you out to dinner." Mr Gardener was tripping over his pyjama bottoms trying to follow us.

"Goodbye Mr Gardener." I closed the door firmly and we jumped into the car.

We called in the surgery on our way to see if there were any new messages. Miss West, the elderly receptionist gazed at Susie in amazement as I introduced her, as did two of the doctors, about to set off on their rounds.

Dr Gallagher senior was still in and I took the opportunity to tell him about Mrs Green who was worried about her husband, an old man with a bad heart who hadn't come up to bed for the last two nights.

"Well, where was he?" he enquired.

"Sleeping in the chair downstairs, and that makes his legs swell up."

"Och! – I thought you meant he was out with a wee floosie!"

I gave up and with all eyes on my student's legs, we left.

Our next visit in North Green was to a young man with a nasty carbuncle on his left buttock.

"Ooh gosh! That's a big one!" Nurse Carlson cried; hardly the most tactful of remarks.

Pus flew in all directions as I removed the dressing.

"Ooh wow! Can I give it a squeeze?"

"Be my guest." I replied

Susie set to work as the patient gnawed his pillow.

"You're cruel you lot," he gasped with feeling as we put on a new dressing. "Why do you have to enjoy it so much?"

"Sorry – but it did have to be done and it'll be much better tomorrow, you'll see," I told him as we left.

We nipped home for a quick sandwich lunch while Susie regaled me with tales of her day out with the Health Visitor. They had visited an old lady who had told the health visitor, Miss Knight, she was being badly treated by the daughter whom she lived with and who didn't really want her.

"She had a bandage on her arm and when Miss Knight asked her why, she said her daughter had bitten her in temper. Miss Knight said, 'Oh I'm sure she hasn't' and the old lady said 'well go on then, take the bandage off and see', and when we did there was a perfect set of teeth marks in her arm and it was all bruised!"

I explained to Susie that as well as 'baby battering' it was possible to come across cases of 'granny battering' or elderly abuse as we called it, and although these were difficult cases to handle, we had to be aware of it and be vigilant.

Susie was still chattering as we got back in the car.

"Then we went to visit another old lady who was nearly ninety years old and her son wanted to put her in a home and sell her house. After Miss Knight talked to her she said she felt a lot better and as we were about to go she said, 'Oh you've been so kind! Before you go will you come upstairs and have a look at my mother?' Well, we looked at each other, like, how **can** she still have a mother? And we followed her upstairs to a huge oil painting of this hideous looking lady dressed in Victorian clothes; her eyes seemed to follow us, really stern she looked. I wouldn't have liked to meet <u>her</u> on a dark night I can tell you. And the old lady said to Miss Knight, 'there you are – isn't she beautiful?' And Miss Knight managed to say 'oh, yes she is' but I was speechless." Susie speechless, I thought in wonder.

We finished our work and I dropped Susie at the purple car. I had set her some home-work and I asked if she'd enjoyed her day.

"Ooh yes!" she said, "especially squeezing that lad's bum!"

I cringed at the unprofessional language of a new generation, but at least she had some enthusiasm, not just looking bored stiff like some of them.

Liz, my next student a few months later was rather different. She appeared to be a very nice girl and showed interest in the patients and their conditions, but most of the time was quiet with an air of sadness about her. On our third day together the reason became apparent, following a visit to a patient dying of a chest disease.

"That's just what my dad's like," said Liz in a small voice I could only just hear. Her father was dying of asbestosis and mesothelioma. Asbestosis was a fairly newly recognized chest disease caused by minute fibres of blue asbestos being inhaled into the lungs where it settled and caused lung disease including mesothelioma, which was malignant, many years – often up to forty years – later.

Asbestos was a fire resistant material used in many buildings, including textile mills, and one in particular in Hebden Bridge had claimed many victims. Our local chest physician had been to the fore-front in describing this condition and presenting and publishing papers, as so many patients had ended up under his care. Unfortunately, treatment was palliative only.

Liz was from Hebden Bridge and most of her family had worked in this mill, now closed, over the last forty years and many of them had contracted the disease which in the end would prove fatal. She had already lost her grandfather and two uncles, and two aunts were also victims. I felt very sorry for my sad little student.

* * *

Simon was not looking forward to my visit – and I was not looking forward to seeing Simon. Circumcisions had never been my favourite cases. Not surprisingly little boys took great exception to this sudden, and in their eyes, quite unwarranted assault on the most delicate part of their anatomy. They arrived home from hospital very sore, having lost a good deal of faith in human nature – and with a permanent hatred of anyone in a blue uniform. To find that one such nurse was determined to follow him even into his own home, to examine and dress the offending part, was an outrage to four year old Simon.

It's usual for a district nurse to enter a home and take command of the situation, but I'd always found, where children were concerned, so much depended on the attitude of the parents. Sensible parents supported the nurse and paid no attention to tears and tantrums, indeed, as a rule there were few tantrums from children of sensible parents. Spoilt children however, screamed and paddied and turned to their distraught, doting mothers for protection from this intruder in the blue dress.

Here Simon was lucky – devoted mummy and daddy were both on hand to protect him – a somewhat genteel couple who obviously preferred to avoid life's unpleasant situations.

"Right then Simon," I said in business-like fashion, "lets put you in a nice warm bath and change the dressing."

"I don't want to go in the bath," wailed Simon.

"He doesn't want to go in the bath," echoed Mummy.

I smiled, what I hoped was a patient smile.

"No of course he doesn't want to go in the bath, Mrs Timpson, but I'm afraid we have to remove the dirty dressing and put on a clean sterile one. Now, shall I go and run the bath or will you?"

Simon, at least, sensed the determination in my voice.

"I don't want to have my dressing changed!" he screamed as his face turned red with rage. I felt sorry for him until his left foot swung out and connected with my shin.

"He doesn't want to have his dressing changed," repeated Daddy.

My patient smile had turned into a grimace with the pain in my shin, and I probably looked half-witted. We stood looking at each other for a moment and I wondered who would make the next move. Simon made the next move. In a split second he changed from a miserable, pathetic infant, into something resembling an enraged orang-outang. He danced round and round the room, jumping on and off the furniture and clinging to the curtains as he passed, screaming "I – DON'T – WANT – TO – GO – IN THE – BATH!"

It was most impressive and I could quite see why Mr and Mrs Timpson had hesitated about forcing him to do so. They had obviously allowed the child to have all his own way from the day he was born, and were now at a loss as to how to control him, even when it was for his own good. I decided to concede round one to Simon.

"Mrs Timpson, I think I'd better leave Simon to calm down, but the dressing has to be changed, otherwise the wound could become infected. I shall call back at two o'clock. Please have Simon sitting in the bath by then." And I left to continue my visits.

I stopped at the clinic as I was passing and made a call to the ward sister at the hospital where Simon had had his minor surgery.

"I just wanted to make it clear it's not my fault if he gets an infection – a reluctant child is one thing, but when the parents are on his side I've got no chance," I moaned.

"Ah! Yes! Well I'm not surprised you've had trouble with that little perisher, he bit Mr Jackson when he did his round."

Mr Jackson was the genitor-urinary surgeon. He could be very arrogant and bad-tempered with patients and nurses, and I had felt like biting him myself at times.

I laughed. "I shouldn't think that improved his temper."

"It didn't – he wrote on the notes – 'This operation would not have been necessary if the parents had taken my advice and gradually stretched the fore-skin'. So he does know what you're up against."

I found that small comfort as I drove back to the Timpson household. It was exactly two o'clock as I walked down the path. I could hear the bath running as I ran upstairs, knocked and walked in. My patient, however, was not in it. He was running naked round the bedroom, doing a repeat performance of his previous party piece, with Mummy and Daddy as the audience. I decided the approach had to be a psychological one.

"Good heavens, Simon! Are you still making a fuss? Matthew Walton across the road didn't cry at all when he had his dressing changed." Simon chose to ignore this remark.

"You'll never be on the rugby team if you're such a softy, will you?"

This struck home, not to Simon, but to Mr Timpson. He made a grab for his son as he ran past, and seizing him, tucked him firmly under his arm.

"I'm sick of this bloody carry-on," he declared, "you're going in the bath!"

Simon kicked and struggled, his face a delicate shade of purple.

"Oh Geoffrey, don't hurt him," wailed Mrs Timpson.

"You've spoilt this child," he yelled at her, "well Sister's right, of course the dressing has to be changed, it's for his own good."

By this time we were all at the top of the stairs. I tested the bath water quickly as Mr Timpson crammed his wriggling, screaming son into it. I had never been squashed into a small bathroom with three other people before, there was no room to move. Simon's screams had an hysterical ring as he splashed his arms wildly and, leaping up, drenched Mr Timpson and I. At this, Mr Timpson's large hand made contact with Simon's left buttock with a resounding crack.

"Oh! Geoffrey!" wailed Mrs Timpson as Mr Timpson turned just in time to see her, face drained of colour, sink to the floor in a dead faint. As he lunged forward to try and catch her, his head struck the wash-basin with a nauseating crunch, and knees buckling, he joined his wife stretched out on the tiles. Simon, in his frantic efforts to get out of the bath, slipped and disappeared under the water. I had only been in the house five minutes and I had laid out the whole family!

I rescued Simon from the watery grave he so richly deserved by pulling out the plug and hauling him to his feet. Fortunately the dirty dressing had floated off in the water and the sight of both parents semi-conscious on the floor silenced him at last. I quickly dried him and applied the dressing.

Mr and Mrs Timpson had by this time come round and were sitting up, Mr Timpson groaning and rubbing a large bump on his head. He looked at me plaintively.

"How often do we have to bath him and change the blasted dressing?"

"At least once a day for a week, I'm afraid," I replied.

"Oh God! We'll never survive it" he groaned, getting to his feet.

"Yes you will because Simon isn't going to make a fuss like this again, are you Simon?" I rather suspected he had been very shocked at the results of his bad behaviour.

I staggered exhausted to my car, hat dripping and knocked awry, dress half soaked, feet squelching in wet shoes – and tomorrow I had to go through it all again.

That evening the phone rang. It was Sue, one of my colleagues.

"Hey, Baines – I've got a student with me tomorrow and I'm short of interesting cases – have you got anything suitable you'd like to pass over?"

"Always glad to help – er – have you got any children to visit?" I asked, feeling slightly wicked.

"Oh no! – that's the trouble, they're nearly all geriatrics. Have you got one to spare?"

"Oh yes! I think I can let you take him, it's a little circumcision on Windsor Avenue –"

* * *

"What a beautiful day it is – I think we're going to enjoy this!" said the voice from the back seat of my car. Three of us, myself and two colleagues from the other end of division 18, were on our way to a refresher course at Grantley Hall near Ripon. Grantley Hall was a minor stately home which had been purchased by West Riding County Council for meetings, study days and courses.

'You speak for yourself' I thought gloomily, thinking about my daughter facing her first day at school without me to take her and bring her home. I'd been foolish enough to mention this big milestone to Miss Burton who had promptly arranged for me to be sent on a refresher course at exactly the same time. I protested to no avail.

"Your family commitments are not my problem Mrs Baines. I'm sure you'll be able to arrange for some Tom, Dick or Harry to look after your daughter for a day or two." The woman was offensive and how often I had wished I had a tape recorder to document what she actually said.

At the end of a long drive, we arrived at Grantley Hall. From the outside it was a beautiful building built in the early seventeen hundreds, with tall leaded windows and pale stonework which reflected the early evening sun. The grounds were magnificent with manicured grass and rhododendrons just at their best.

We found we were in a small dormitory of four beds with screens round each bed. We wondered who our companion would be as we unpacked, until the door opened and a rather mousey woman in a tweed suit walked in and we found out. It was none other than Miss Denham, the midwife who was Miss Burton's companion in life. They lived together on my patch.

We set off to the sitting room to report in and have a cup of tea.

"It's like being at boarding school and sharing a dorm with the school sneak!" I muttered gloomily, thinking about Miss Denham.

"It's thrown a spanner in my works," said Helen, "I hadn't intended sleeping in this place after tonight."

Anne and I looked at her in amazement. "Where are you thinking of sleeping?" Anne asked, "we're here for four nights aren't we?"

"My – er – boyfriend has a flat in Ripon and I shall be there for three nights."

Anne and I couldn't believe our ears but it turned out Helen, a farmer's wife with four children, had been having an ardent affair with a chicken feed salesman for years. This opportunity was too good to miss until Miss B's sneak had been billeted with us.

"You two'll have to cover for me," said Helen, "I'll stick a pillow down the bed so it looks like I'm there and keep the curtains round my cubicle."

"And what if she calls on you to borrow some curlers or something?" I asked, "and what when you're not there in the morning?"

"Oh – you'll think of something," said Helen.

"Well don't blame us when you're hauled into the lion's den next week!" said Anne.

After an evening meal we all filed into the lecture room. Our first speaker was a G.P from a group of doctors whose surgeries were near the A1 in North Yorkshire. This area was a long way from the nearest accident and emergency centre and these G.P's were willing to attend road accidents on the A1 and give first aid of a high standard to increase survival rates.

He talked about their work in general and he demonstrated some of the latest equipment and in particular he wanted to show us an inflatable splint which he himself had designed. It was made of tough plastic, brightly coloured like children's armbands. He asked for a volunteer from the audience and a rather attractive, tall blonde in her early thirties jumped up onto the stage. The splint was fitted over one of her legs un-inflated and unfortunately the valve landed right at the top in a rather embarrassing position.

"And what happens now?" asked our colleague looking distinctly uncomfortable. The doctor ignored her and turning to his students declared, "I shall now inflate the splint."

"You'll do no such thing!" said the nurse.

Being arrogant he ignored her again and to our astonishment his head disappeared between her legs. There was a resounding crack as the nurse struck him across his face. He looked rather flustered as he jumped to his feet.

"Well, I'm sure you all get the general idea – of – er – inflatable – er splints and their ease of use."

"Depends who's using them," said our nurse in a loud voice as she pulled the splint off and went back to her place.

And so, our first evening finished, followed by a stampede for the bar. I got in the queue to phone home. I couldn't wait to hear about Lucy's first day at school. It was a small private junior school and Lucy was starting in the nursery class at three, mornings only. A friend had kindly agreed to take her and bring her home again at lunch time. Marjorie assured me Lucy had taken to it like a duck to water and had gone into the class without a backward glance. Picking her up again Marjorie found her to be a changed child. Clutching a strangely shaped lump of papier maché, in a posh cut glass accent she said, "Look Auntie Marjorie, I've made a brontosaurus."

It was a relief to settle down in our strange dormitory knowing that all was well at home.

The next day a young labour M.P., who was a solicitor came to lecture us on 'Nursing and the Law,' which made us very aware that things were changing, people were becoming more litigious, and we were likely to be sued if we made mistakes. Sadly this young M.P., was killed in a road accident a few years later.

We were privileged to have a lecture from Dame Cicely Saunders, who had travelled up from London to talk to us about developments in terminal care through the hospice movement.

Dame Cicely had trained as a nurse and then trained as a doctor, which gave her a unique view on patient care from both the nursing and medical aspects.

The care of the dying was not being well managed, particularly in hospitals. The principle of hospice care was symptom control, particularly pain control. Dame Cicely was a truly inspiring speaker and she made an enormous impression on us. It was so exciting to think we were going to change things for the better.

For the next three nights, Anne and I tried to cover up the fact that Helen had gone off on the razzle. Miss Denham gave no sign that she had noticed she was missing but short of saying good morning and good night to her we had very little conversation. She was well aware that living with Miss B. put her in a different category to the rest of us.

On our last evening, to our surprise, Helen rolled in after midnight and somewhat the worse for wear. The chicken feed salesman's car had broken down and Helen had decided she'd rather walk back to Grantley Hall than walk to Ripon. Anne and I woke up as she tripped over the end of Miss Denham's bed and a loud "bugger it!" rent the air. We pushed her into her own cubicle and on to her bed. She was giggling and hiccoughing now as we pulled her shoes off and covered her with her quilt, trying to shush her in vain.

As I crept back to my own little cosy corner, Miss Denham's curtains parted and the somewhat ghastly sight of her head appeared, face covered in white cream and hair in curlers and a thick net.

"Is everything alright?" she asked, "What's all the noise?"

"Oh yes, Helen just er slipped coming back from the bathroom, that's all" I replied.

"Oh, she's decided to sleep here tonight has she?" – the ghastly head disappeared. She hadn't been fooled for a minute!

A subdued Helen travelled back with us next morning. "I've decided to chuck him," she confided. "His flat is a tip and he smells of his damned chicken feed."

I never found out if Miss B. sent for her or not.

Chapter 6

Changes were happening in most areas of my life in the early seventies. Our marriage had been in difficulty for some time. Now Rob and I decided to split up. Lucy and I stayed in the cottage. We tried our best to protect her from the hurt of seeing her parents separate but I shall draw a veil over this part of my life.

Work was my saviour and it kept me going. Spending all day with people who were worse off than myself made me count my blessings.

Edna was about to retire. Her husband had died the previous winter and now her precious animals meant more to her than ever. Her menagerie had reduced to Bertie, a ginger tom, and Jet and Sandy, her two dogs. Bertie had chronic sinusitis and his party piece was to walk into the middle of a room and do an enormous sneeze, covering everyone within range with green snot. Jet was a black collie with long, very fine black hairs which got into everything, particularly my sandwiches if I popped in for lunch. Sandy was a golden Labrador with wanderlust, usually connected to his love life.

"If you see Sandy on your travels bring him home kid, he's disappeared again," she would say on her day off as I set off for Queenstown.

Occasionally, I did spot him, trotting along miles from home following the scent of some lady love. I would have to stop and heave him into the car, until one day, not having looked too closely, I returned the wrong labrador.

"Hey kid! That's not Sandy!" said a puzzled Edna, and I had to take an outraged dog back to where I'd found him.

Our work load, particularly the eighty-five plus age range, was gradually increasing as people started living longer and these were the most dependent. All over the country district nursing itself was changing from one nurse being responsible for a geographic area, to being attached to general practitioner's surgeries.

This meant we actually travelled further, going anywhere within the limits of the practice, so now we all crossed over each others previous patches and you could have several nurses visiting on the same street. This took a bit of getting used to but as each surgery now had its own nurse, communication and co-operation became better. This way of working was thought to be in the patients' best interest and most of us welcomed it.

The old way of working from home also fell out of favour and we moved into offices in health centres and clinics. We called into our clinics at nine a.m, two p.m and five p.m., before going off duty. With Edna retiring, I had new colleagues.

Spending so much time calling in to clinics could be tiresome and it had a lot to do with a policing type of nurse management which wanted to keep tabs on us at all times, and was terrified we might finish early and go home. On the other hand at least the phone at home didn't ring constantly and we didn't feel as if we were on duty all the time, but gone was taking the rough with the smooth; perish the thought we should have any smooth!

This change came hand in hand with an obsession with meetings and we were constantly dashing through our work to get to meetings with several tiers of nurse management. Courses and study days became more frequent and although it was obviously important to keep abreast of developments, what with going into clinics and surgeries, meetings and study days and extra paper work, we began to wonder when we'd find time to care for our patients.

Some developments were however, a great and necessary step forward. Nursing auxiliaries began to be employed and I was given first one, then two to do a lot of the tasks that did not necessarily require a qualified sister. Equipment improved and became more readily available and we at last had a plentiful supply of sterile dressings and instruments. The days of boiling up instruments in the home were long gone.

Having worked mainly for the Galbraith practice for years, I was happy to become attached to them. Midwives and health visitors also became attached so that team working was the new approach. Gradually care of patients in the community was being dragged into the twentieth century – even though it was nearly the twenty first.

* * *

After our re-shuffle of patients following G.P attachment, Mr Sutcliffe at Southowram, a diabetic on insulin, became one of my first visits of the day. He was a taciturn old gentleman who sat almost on top of his open fire which unfortunately belched smoke and small particles of soot into the room. On top of that, he smoked a pipe filled with the most foul smelling tobacco, which meant I could just about make him out through the smog. Every few minutes he would have a coughing fit followed by spitting the results into the fire. He wore a heavy duty suit with waistcoat and a thick flannelette shirt winter and summer, plus huge black lace up boots.

I would say a cheery good morning and ask him to get ready for his injection. He would wait until I was standing next to him, syringe ready in receiver, before beginning laboriously to extricate himself from these garments, which drove me mad. By the look of the shiny suit and grubby shirt I suspected he had been wearing the same thing for years and as he was a widower there was no sign of the house being cleaned either. He refused to have a home help.

"What for?" he would ask indignantly, "leave me alone – I'm right enough!"

One morning I arrived to a locked door. On peering in at the dirty window, Mr Sutcliffe was nowhere in view and the fire was unlit. I spent a few minutes calling through the letterbox and banging on the door without result. I decided to call on my next nearest patient and pop back.

As I drew up outside the Johnsons' I was amazed to see Mrs Johnson standing on the doorstep in her nightie with her hair in curlers.

"Let me in Harold, please!" she was wailing through the letterbox.

Oh great! Another locked door and another patient I couldn't get at.

Mr and Mrs Johnson had had a long marriage during which Mrs Johnson had worn the trousers. He had been henpecked and under the thumb, but since his recent stroke his personality had changed somewhat; he now fought back and took delight in thwarting her at every opportunity. We looked through the window. Mr Johnson , wearing nothing but his night shirt, grinned and waved at us.

"Please Harold, let me in" begged Mrs Johnson. The reply was in the form of a rude gesture with two fingers.

"Harold! You stupid bugger, open this bloody door or I'll call the police!" Mrs Johnson's face was a snarling mass of anger pressed up against the window. Another rude gesture, this time with both hands, as he danced a little jig, chuckling with glee.

Mrs Johnson was crying tears of rage.

"I only stepped out to get the milk and he pushed me and locked the door. He's done this because I have an appointment at the hospital and I'll miss it if he doesn't let me in."

I left her, almost blue with cold, going to a neighbour's to call the police, whilst I drove back to see if Mr Sutcliffe was up. The door was still locked and he was nowhere to be seen. As I shouted through the letterbox again his neighbours at both sides came out.

"Sorry about the noise," I said, "but I must get in."

The lady on the left pulled a pessimistic face.

"He's always up early as a rule – I bet he's dead." She looked almost hopeful.

"Mary, his wife, was a lovely person and he treated her like a slave, bossing and bullying, and when she was taken ill she collapsed on the floor and he just left her

94

there for two days! **Two days**! I sent for the ambulance – not him. It won't bother me if he's dead!"

I decided to go back to the Johnsons' and borrow their policeman. By now, neighbours and a few passers-by with nothing better to do, were gathered on the pavement at both venues to watch the goings on. A disappointingly small, ginger haired young man who looked about twelve years old, in a police constable's uniform was negotiating with Mr Johnson along the lines of – 'you open the door and I won't have to break it down and arrest you for disturbing the peace.'

The door was unlocked by a subdued Mr Johnson and I explained I would be back soon but I needed the policeman round the corner.

"Show's over folks, go home," said my weedy ginger rescuer to the small crowd, but they'd cottoned on to a bit more drama in the offing and they followed us back to Mr Sutcliffe's.

The loquacious neighbour greeted us. "He hasn't appeared – I bet he's dead!"

The policeman tried some half hearted shouting through the letterbox, accompanied by banging on the door.

"It's no good doing that – we've all tried that," said the neighbour.

"Stand back please Madam," said my policeman as he started to kick the bottom of the old wooden panelled door, accompanied by cheers from some rag-a-muffin children. My suggestion that he was supposed to run at it with his shoulder like they did on Z-cars was met with a withering look. Suddenly the door started to give and as it flew open Mr Sutcliffe was revealed coming downstairs in his night shirt.

"Are you alright?" the police officer and I chorused together.

"Of course I'm alright! Why shouldn't I be? I just slept in that's all. What a fuss – and look at my door!" He was incandescent with rage.

"We thought you were dead," said the neighbour, looking disappointed.

The policeman stayed whilst I gave the insulin as there was a fair chance Mr Sutcliffe would murder me. For the next few days he tried to swipe me every time I gave his injection. Still, for the good people of Southowram there hadn't been such excitement since World War Two when a German bomber had dropped his load by mistake and killed two cows.

* * *

"Sister Baines, I see your doctors never leave messages on your nursing notes." Miss Burton, pouncing on me as I called in to the Health Department, had found something else to complain about. Message communication sheets were left in our patients homes and sent in to the Health Department with our nursing notes when the case was finished.

"Why do you think that is Sister?" I felt like saying I had no b—- idea and cared even less. I was sure they thought it was a waste of time when they saw me every day.

"Discuss it with them will you?" Damn!

Dutifully next morning I asked if they could write something occasionally just to keep Miss B. off my back. This was greeted by guffaws of laughter and a few suggestions as to what they could write. They had little time for Miss Burton or Dr Scrimshaw, alias Pansy Potter.

For the next few weeks I found a succession of inappropriate or even lurid messages here and there, thankfully usually where the patient was unable to read them. Now I had the extra job of re-writing or re-arranging the notes to make them acceptable to Miss B. and the office lot at the Health Department.

Now that we had staff to manage as well as our patients and districts, it was decided by someone at the Department of Health, that district nursing sisters should go on a course: First Line Management for Nurses; and when my turn came I was sent to Huddersfield Polytechnic, now University.

We were a mixture of community staff and hospital ward sisters and to some extent it was a refreshing change from the usual frenzied round of daily life. We did lots of group working and bandying round of ideas and opinions, which was felt had little connexion with how to manage staff. We listened to various lecturers, the most interesting of whom was a senior bacteriologist who told us that antibiotics had been over prescribed for years, that bacterial resistance was growing, and in the near future more patients would die as we ran out of new antibiotics. All this came to pass exactly as predicted.

In order to study a management structure different to our own, we were sent in various groups on different days to spend a day at Storthes Hall, a large mental institution miles out in the country.

A new era of enlightened thinking regarding mental illness was about to result in the closure of these huge hospitals as it was realised that many of the patients, locked away from society for thirty or forty years, should never have been there in the first place, and that there had to be a better way of caring for people, many of whom were merely simple and inadequate or had learning difficulties. Meanwhile, these huge, almost self sufficient communities behind high walls in acres of grounds, were still with us.

My fellow students and I arrived in the main entrance hall and were met by the deputy matron who gave us a pep talk about the place before allocating us to a different ward each. I was asked to present myself at 56B, a locked ward for psychotic long stay patients.

As I plodded along miles of bleak corridors I heard feet running in the distance but rapidly approaching behind me. I turned and saw a rather large clumsy man who was waving at me to stop. There was no one else in sight and I felt somewhat wary as he drew level, puffing for breath.

"I'm ready Aunty Betty! – are we going home now?" he gasped.

"Er – sorry – I think you've made a mistake." I stammered.

"You're not my Aunty Betty are you?" His face crumpled and to my horror a big tear rolled down his cheek. As I walked on he sank to the floor in a big heap and put his head in his hands. I felt dreadful I wasn't his Aunty Betty.

Arriving at the ward I pressed the bell and a male nurse with a huge bunch of keys let me in. I told him about the incident with the strange man as we introduced ourselves.

"Oh! – that's Wilfred – he's been looking for his Aunty Betty for thirty years but he's harmless. Anyway, come and read Hobson's Choice."

In the middle of the ward a circle of patients sat holding scripts of the famous play. George, the charge nurse, introduced me and I smiled round the group. They regarded me warily except for Sid who waved and blew me a kiss.

"I like your jumper. Do you like my jumper?" he asked gazing at my chest.

"Thank you Sid!" said George, "concentrate on the play please."

"What size bra are you wearing?" Sid didn't want to concentrate on anything but their new visitor.

"Enough Sid!" George was getting ratty.

"Alright – keep your hair on!" Sid turned his chair round and sat with his back to us sulking.

George ignored him. "Right off we go. Pam can you read Hobson? Bert, you start."

Bert read his lines slowly and carefully until we were interrupted by an old lady, eighty five if she was a day, pushing a trolley of coffee and biscuits.

"Hurry up Violet," said George somewhat ungratefully, "we've just started reading."

Violet handed round the cups of coffee and nudged me on the shoulder.

"I'm going home today." I smiled at her.

"My mother's coming for me." George's eyes met mine and he shook his head. Violet trundled off happily and we started to read again.

I was in the middle of a long speech when an old lady opposite got up and walked to the middle of the circle. Waving her arms as if to music only she could hear, she started to take her clothes off. No one batted an eyelid until she was down to her vest, then Bert decided he'd had enough.

"For heaven's sake Effie sit down! We've seen it all before!"

Effie picked up her bra and wound it round Bert's neck, whereupon Bert's temper snapped and he started to chase Effie down the ward. Two of the others carried on reading their parts in happy oblivion.

Later on, play abandoned, when George had restored order, Effie had re-robed and Bert was playing 'Oh I do like to be beside the sea-side' on a piano in the corner, I asked George what was the point of the play reading.

"It's all about trying to get them to behave in socially acceptable ways in society," he told me.

Over lunch, only marred by the two mile trek to the dining room, we shared our experiences. Susie had offered to help an old man, dressed as a vicar, to cut his toenails and was called a harlot, a jezebel and a strumpet for her pains.

Back on the ward, we sat in George's office while he explained the principles of care and the management structure of the unit. We were just about to enjoy a cup of tea when an alarming commotion broke out, seemingly in the kitchen. Two female patients, brandishing spoons, no knives allowed on the ward, were fighting over a custard cream.

Leaving George at the end of the shift he said he'd enjoyed my visit and was sorry it had been such a quiet, uneventful day! We gathered in the car park for our journey back to Huddersfield. All agreed how sad it was so many people were incarcerated for years in such depressing surroundings but we didn't know who to feel most sorry for, the patients or the staff.

"There but for the grace of God," said Susie. Amen to that.

* * *

Mr and Mrs Carter had been happily married for over forty years and Mr Harry Carter had just retired when Connie began to be very forgetful. At first they put this down to anno domini as Harry felt his memory was not as sharp as it had been, but then Connie started doing strange things and the problem could no longer be ignored.

Returning from the shops one day Connie was nowhere to be seen until Harry spotted her at the bottom of the garden running the vacuum cleaner round the lawn.

"Whatever are you doing love?" Harry asked, but his heart felt to be sinking into his boots. "The lawn's my job anyway."

"Well you haven't done it very well have you? There's all these brown bits all over the place." Connie pushed her Hoover roughly back and forward over the leaves. "I can't understand why it's not picking them up."

"Well, it's not plugged in!" Harry started but in the ludicrousness of the situation explanations like that were pointless, crazy, irrelevant.

"You'll have me as daft as you next," he said and as he manoeuvred her into the kitchen still clutching the vacuum, he noticed Mrs Hoggard's curtains twitching next door.

After a cup of tea and a nice sit down Connie seemed to be back to her old self and the rest of the day passed without incident. Two days later Harry found Connie had put the washing into the oven, turned on high, and his two best pairs of leather shoes were clattering round in the washing machine. It was time to visit the doctor.

Connie sat looking sulky as she felt fine and didn't know why on earth they needed to visit the surgery. The doctor looked kindly at her and asked her what the date was.

"I don't know why you're asking me, you've got a calendar right in front of you." She snapped. Round one to Connie. He tried again. "How old are you now?"

"Old enough to know better than sit here answering silly questions," she replied. Harry groaned. "Just tell the doctor Connie, don't be silly." She glared at them both in silence. The doctor gave up. "In view of what you've told me Mr Carter, I'll refer her to the Geriatrician anyway."

A few weeks later the Geriatrician fared rather better with his diagnostic questions as Connie was in a much better mood.

"Can you tell me who the Prime Minister is please Mrs Carter?"

"Well I'm surprised you don't know that," Connie replied, "a man with your education; its Mr Churchill!"

"What's the date, please?"

"Don't you know that either? Its 1944 – it might be March – I'm not sure which day though – doesn't that barometer thing tell you, on your desk?"

Sister took Connie off for a cup of tea while the consultant explained to Harry that Connie was probably suffering from Alzheimer's disease and that there was very little that could be done. Their doctor would keep an eye on things and he would see Connie again from time to time. Perhaps the district nurse would be needed at some future stage.

"Well, what can she do?" Harry asked, then wished he hadn't.

"She may become incontinent I'm afraid, and the nurse will be able to help and advise management, of course if you reach a stage where you can't cope we can consider a bed here at the hospital."

That evening Harry sat with tears pouring down his face.

"Whatever are you crying for love? – did I burn the dinner again?"

Harry shook his head and blew his nose.

"Well cheer up then, my mother's coming round soon and you don't want her to see you crying." Her mother had been dead for twenty five years.

A few months later I was called in. A kind neighbour who felt she could cope, had taken Connie with her to the shops, giving me the chance to sit with a distraught Harry and hear his story.

"I don't know what to do – I don't want her to go into hospital but she's driving me mad. We have these circular conversations – she asks about all her brothers and sisters and how old they are now and when are we going to see them and if I tell her they're all dead she cries, and then she forgets why she's crying and starts again at the beginning. It can go on like that for hours."

I made us both a cup of tea and just listened and listened as it all poured out. They only had one son and sadly he had gone to Australia ten years previously. They had never seen their two grandchildren.

"Most of our friends have stopped visiting or inviting us to them as they don't know how to cope with Connie. The last time friends came round she said, "When are they going Harry? – I don't know who they are anyway." So that was the last of a couple we used to go on holiday with. People don't understand unless it's happened to them. She gets up sometimes at all hours of the night and once I didn't hear her – I'm a bit deaf now – and she'd wandered into the village in her nightie and a policeman brought her home, only because he knew her – a local lad – as otherwise she couldn't have told him where she lived. I'm on watch twenty four hours a day. She does the most maddening things and then I shout at her and she cries and I feel a right swine. Sometimes I take her for a run in the car in the afternoon. Those are the best times; she loves going out; mind you, she insists on wearing an old purple hat with a feather in it and she waves to people like she's the Queen."

Some of Harry's tension had dissipated with being able to talk to someone and he was laughing now.

"One day we stopped by a field of sheep in the country, to eat our sandwiches. She looked at them and said, 'I've always liked those.' I said, 'do you know what they are?' and she said scornfully, 'Of course I do, do you think I'm daft? They're – you know – jumpers, cardigans, knit ones, purl ones.' Harry chuckled and shook his head. "I suppose she was on the right lines. "

Shortly after that Connie did start to be incontinent and this made Harry's life much harder. I provided pads and various other aids and asked Sheila, one of my auxiliary nurses to visit to help with bathing but it felt like precious little. When I popped in Harry was tearful again.

"I'm so frightened." he kept saying.

"Frightened of what Harry?" I asked gently. Then out it came.

"I love her but she wears me down and I never get a moments peace. She asks me the same things over and over and I'm frightened I'll completely lose my temper and I'm frightened I'll hit her. There! I've said it at last."

He put his head in his hands. For once I didn't know what to say or how to comfort him.

"Would you like us to try and get her a bed in hospital? You could visit every day."

"No! – no! – she'd die in there – locked up with others as bad as herself. We've never been parted."

"I'm just as concerned about you as Connie, you know. We have to think about you as well." I patted Harry's shoulder.

I told Dr Craig everything but unless he would let her go there was nothing we could do.

A few months later the situation resolved itself when Harry collapsed and died of a heart attack and Connie had to go into a nursing home. Many of the friends who'd deserted them turned up for the funeral. Connie wore her favourite purple hat with the feather and waved at passers-by from the cortege. Her son came over from Australia and escorted her into church. In a moment of quiet when the organ had stopped and just before the vicar spoke, Connie said in a loud voice. –

"Who's in the coffin?"

"It's Dad," said her son, appalled.

"Whose dad? – its not my dad – we buried him years ago."

"No – it's Dad! My dad! Your husband Harry."

"Harry? It's not Harry, he's at home making the dinner. Anyway, who are you?"

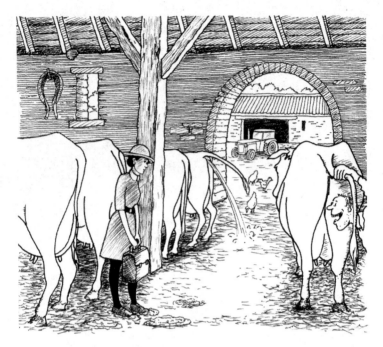

Chapter 7

"You see he was gassed in the trenches, he's always had a bad chest." Josh's wife told me. I seemed to hear this so often when I was nursing the veterans who'd fought in the First World War. What a nightmare it must have been. The wives would often tell me things but usually the old men didn't want to talk about it. Apart from bringing back terrible memories they felt no words could possibly convey the horror of it. My father who had been a glider pilot in Normandy on D-Day and had fought at Arnhem in the Second World War, would often say, "you can watch all the war films you like, you still won't have a clue what battle is like."

Many of the old men had strange scars or huge hollows in their back or chest muscles where they'd been hit by shrapnel and many had lost limbs. I knew when they told me they'd got a 'Blighty' – it meant an injury bad enough to be sent home; as the song said, 'Take me back to dear old Blighty!'

Josh was different in that, if he was in the mood, he did want to talk about the war and many of his stories were humorous as well as heart breaking, but most of all he wanted to talk about his beloved horses. He and his father before him, were the local blacksmiths and Josh's job after he was called up in 1914 into the cavalry, was to look after the horses.

He and Mary lived on a small holding where they'd brought up five children and had kept horses all their married lives, until Josh's health had broken down and all their animals had to go. He missed the horses desperately.

The old cottage they lived in looked as if it hadn't been updated in any way since it was built. There was no electricity, hence no washing machine, and Mary cooked on the range heated by their open fire, and they used oil lamps for lighting. They had no bathroom but did have a flush toilet out in the yard. The house was bitterly cold and damp in winter, so they had brought their bed downstairs which to them meant they could keep warm and have the pleasure of each others company at all times instead of Josh being upstairs in bed.

My first visit was nearly my last. I asked where the kitchen was to wash my hands and was directed to a heavy door with an old fashioned metal sneck. Opening it, some instinct made me hesitate. It was a very dark room and as my eyes adjusted to the gloom I could see it was more of a cellar down a flight of six steps!

"Oh and mind the steps love!" Mary's warning was a bit late as I'd nearly stepped into thin air. Josh needed my attention to dress his left heel. He'd left his right leg "somewhere on the Somme,' he liked to tell me. Sometimes his false leg made his stump sore and his left heel had been badly damaged by a bullet. After all these years it would still swell and discharge pus from time to time.

"Ah well! I wouldn't put it past those Jerrys to put poison on the bullets. There was no end to how low they'd stoop!" Mary held Josh's leg while I firmly bandaged it. He suddenly kicked out involuntarily.

"Whoa Josh! – whoa there!" Mary had often held horses' legs for him in the smithy and she still used the same language.

"I'm trying to woman! Stop tickling me foot!"

Opposite Josh's bed was a rather amateurish oil painting of a young man in army uniform holding his rifle. "That was our Wally," said Josh, "he were't third son me mother lost."

He nodded towards his wife. "Mary lost two brothers."

We fell into a routine where I would visit twice a week and after attending to Josh I would have a cup of tea and one of Mary's delicious scones, and listen to one of Josh's war stories, usually about his horses.

"Aye them poor horses – many had to be shot because they sank up to their bellies in the mud – no way of getting them out you see – but they were the lucky ones – many lay dying trapped in the wire with no one to tend them; we were too busy fighting for our lives. We used to get them under cover when we could and me and my pal Herbie would sleep with them – it were warmer than in a trench!"

"What happened to Herbie?," I asked one day.

"God only knows! He were leading two horses on duck boards when Jerry started up a heavy bombardment. No one ever saw him again! Blown to smithereens and the horses." He would fall silent and Mary and I knew better than to try to cheer him up with some facile remark.

The days when he preferred his funny stories made happier tea breaks, like the time a visiting Colonel was sitting behind the lines, in a wooden toilet block when a blast from a stray shell blew away the makeshift 'thunder box', as Josh called it, to reveal the Colonel in full view with his trousers round his ankles. Josh always told me this story as if I'd never heard it before and he would laugh until his bed frame rattled and tears rolled down his cheeks.

One morning, as I stopped the car in the yard, Mary came to meet me shaking her head.

"Oh! I'm glad you've come, he'll not have the doctor. I don't know what to do."

Josh was propped up in bed, grey and clammy, eyes closed, and fighting for breath.

"'Allo lass!" He managed a smile as I sponged his face. He stared past my shoulder.

"There's Prince and Jessie come back to see me."

I looked at Mary. "Two of his horses in the war," she whispered.

Tears poured down his face and he became very agitated. "I couldn't look after them properly," he gasped and coughed. "They did everything for us – ferried the wounded," he coughed again, "pulled the guns; they were so faithful," he lay back for a minute then sat up again and clutched at my arm. "We couldn't even get them enough food and water!"

"Now Josh – you must put this out of your mind – it was so long ago and I'm sure you did your best." I tried to soothe him. He looked at me with such anguish on his face.

"But it wasn't enough lass, don't you understand? I can't forgive meself."

"You're very poorly Josh. You really need to go into hospital. Some oxygen would help your breathing."

"Nay lass," he gasped, "I'll stop here, me times up," he paused for breath, "I've had a lot longer than most of me mates, I reckon I'm going to join me leg." He lay back and closed his eyes.

I left Mary holding his hand, promising I'd let his doctor know and I'd come back in an hour or two. When I got back he was lying flat on the bed; his struggle was over. Mary was sitting nearby in her rocking chair.

"The doctor came and gave him an injection to make him more comfortable," she told me, "he went to sleep and that was it."

Tears were running down her face. I stayed until her son and daughter arrived and then I slipped away.

* * *

It was without doubt the worst case of burns I had ever seen. The young man had turned up on my patch, living in a Council flat, his rent paid by Social Security. He had been discharged to my area by the burns unit at Pinderfields Hospital in Wakefield, after a two month stay. His legs were thin and very scarred from the top of his thighs down. He also had patches of healed scarring on his chest, arms and back. Pinderfields had no doubt saved his life.

"What on earth happened to you?" I asked as I examined him.

"Beckwith Festival," was the monosyllabic reply.

Almost on the moors near Saddleworth, at the very edge of our area, a local farmer had decided to make some money by holding a pop festival. Young people had descended from all over the country to see their favourite rock and pop artists, wallow in the mud which always accompanies such gatherings, get rat-arsed on drugs and alcohol, copulate, and generally cause as much trouble for the locals, the emergency services, and anyone within earshot, as possible.

"Yes, but what did you actually do to get into this state?" I asked again. He looked at me impatiently, tired of telling his story.

"In tent, stoned, lighting spliff, dropped match in sleeping bag. Whoosh!"

Whoosh indeed, I thought as I dressed his stick-like legs with the latest state-of-the-art and highly expensive treatment and bandages provided by the hospital. A few weeks later, his burns almost healed, he disappeared, probably in search of another pop concert.

Val, the girl on whose patch the concert had been held, was full of stories of the goings on and how she'd had to go up to the field with one of her doctors to various problems.

We were eating a quick snack lunch in the sitting room at the health department before a meeting. Mary, one of the midwives was listening. "You lot don't know when you're well off – at least you didn't have to go to a delivery."

"Crikey! Did you have to deliver a baby in a tent?"

"No, the farmer let the mum move into an unused cottage on his land so at least I had electricity and running water. The mum absolutely refused to go into hospital. She was with a bunch of hippies who'd driven up in a wreck of a camper van and when I arrived they were sitting in a circle on the floor, chanting and rattling some sort of beans in tins and they were all naked!

Mum, and presumably the father, were on the bed, both naked. I tried to throw the bean rattlers out but they ignored me. Anyway, baby duly arrived to the sound of beans and chants. I kept my clothes on, and when I came back later in the day, they'd all beggared off in their campervan!"

It was weeks before we all got over the excitement of the pop festival and its impact on the local health services, in all its manifestations, but you could say it livened up a dull world.

* * *

The farmyard was deserted except for a few chickens and a scruffy dog chained to the wall, as I pulled my car in at the side of a milking shed. I just haven't time for this today I thought, grabbing my nursing bag from the seat. Visits to farms often took up considerable time since, unless the patients were bedridden, the house was often locked and I had to spend time searching through buildings or even fields, looking for my client.

This morning was a particularly busy one as my colleague was on holiday and the caseload was almost double in number.

The farmhouse looked dirty and in a state of disrepair but this was not unusual – farmers preferred to invest money in stock and equipment and their homes were last on their list of priorities. I knocked and tried the door of the farmhouse – it was open. Inside was a long dismal passage with a stone floor and walls covered in brown gloss paint.

Down the centre of the passage, at varying intervals, were little mounds of dog dirt. I picked my way round them and entered a large and very old-fashioned kitchen. Warmth came from a huge Aga cooker, which reassured me that some human being had stood in this place within the not too distant past.

I called out "Hello," but heard only silence in return. Progressing through the house I entered room after room looking for my patient. Most of the rooms were in darkness with curtains drawn. A fusty damp smell pervaded the atmosphere. Finally in a small bedroom at the back of the house, I found her. Miss Hall, I had been told, was the farmer's sister who had come out of hospital the previous day, and required calcium injections due to a bone deficiency.

She was sound asleep – a large mound in the bed in the darkened room. I drew back the curtains and light entered the dull little cell. A very full chamber pot reposed in the centre of a peg rug. Cardboard boxes, rusty milk crates and papier-mâché egg cartons littered the corner opposite the bed. Old clothes were heaped on every available flat surface. The old lady slept on, amid the chaos. I gave her shoulder a shake and instantly she sat up staring at me. She was quite startling in appearance, with an enormous mis-shapen head, which was almost bald. She looked remarkably like Humpty-Dumpty.

"Good morning, Miss Hall, I've come to give you your injection."

She gazed at me uncomprehendingly and an inarticulate sound came from her mouth. I tried again.

"Have you got your letter from the hospital, and the injections?"

"I can't hear you, you know," she said in the strange voice used by the deaf, who communicate without hearing their own sounds.

Blast! I thought, now I'll have to go on a man hunt round the farm, wondering what had made me think I would escape it. I signalled my intentions to her and she seemed to understand. I picked up my bag and avoiding the overflowing chamber pot and the doggy mess in the hall, I charged back into the yard. Ten precious minutes had already passed. I decided to try the mistle first, since I could hear the cows were still in there.

"Hello! – is anyone here?" I called as I stepped crossly into the middle of two rows of cows.

Most of their heads turned in curiosity to survey the incongruous sight of a district nurse in spotless pristine uniform, complete with hat, leather bag, and black shoes and stockings, standing in the middle of their warm, steaming cowpats.

"Hello there!" A large red face appeared round the backside of the third cow on the left.

"Good morning!" I snapped, as if trying to convey to him I didn't have all day. "I'm Sister Baines, the district nurse," and there I stood, badges and buckles gleaming, in all my officious glory.

"Aa ya now?" he said, moving out from behind the cow. "Well, let's 'ave a look at ye then – ah've nivver sin a district nuss 'afore." He walked all round me slowly, taking in every detail. I felt like the prize bull at the Great Yorkshire Show.

"Well, you look reeght nice, young lady, and what have you come to see me for? – I'm not expectin!" He patted his tummy and roared with laughter at his own joke, one I had heard a million times before.

"I've come to give your sister her injection, Mr Hall."

"Oh aye! Sadie – ah'd forgotten about 'er. I'll tek ye across in a minute, when Daisy's finished milkin." He slapped the nearest cow on her flank. "She's allus last is Daisy, thinks we've got all the time in the world – ony 'ow, it's nice to 'ave a visitor to talk to."

I tried to hide my exasperation.

"Well actually Mr Hall, I am rather busy – if you could just tell me where the injections are I can get on with it and leave you to your milking."

"Aye well, – I don't know about that lass, ya see t'sister on t'ward did give me a little box but I understood as they were pills for Sadie's rheumatics."

"No – I think they'll be my box of injections."

"Oh!" his face fell, "I were 'oping as they were pills, as I were goin' to try 'em for **my** rheumatics."

I looked at him aghast. "Mr Hall, you can't take medication that has been prescribed for another patient, especially when you haven't the faintest idea what it's for!"

"Aay – we don't fuss in our family lass – it's share and share alike 'ere, – what's good for one is good for t'others like." He laughed. The telephone began to ring. There was a large bell which must have rivalled that of the fire station, on the wall over the back door.

"Ye see we've nivver 'eld much wi' doctors – allus treated oursels like – whenever we could." Still the telephone rang. We strolled slowly across the yard.

"Except for specialists that is – specialists is a different matter. D'you know?" he said, stopping to impart the privileged information, "ah've sin every specialist in Bradford and they still don't know what's up wi'me. Ah've baffled 'em I 'ave – baffled 'em!"

I was baffled too, as to how I was ever going to treat this case and get on to the next. The telephone finally gave up in disgust.

"Eee!" said Mr Hall, "will yer look at that now –some folk won't wait a minute will they? Now, where was I? Oh aye! I was telling ye about me ailments wasn't I?"

How can I stop you? I thought, looking at him. A healthier looking man I had never seen. He was built like a rugby prop-forward, with a glowing round face and hands like shovels. The hairs on his chest were bursting through the gaps in his shirt. By this time, we had actually reached the door. A small collie dog came fussing round his huge feet – obviously the offspring of the one chained to the wall.

"Mr Hall, there's dog dirt all down the passage." At least it was an attempt to change the subject.

"Is there now?" he laughed and kicked gently at the affectionate dog. "See Cromwell, ye dirty little bugger, tha maunt do that when t' district nuss is comin, – she dun't like it!"

I followed him into the living room in search of the box from the hospital. The mess was indescribable. Used crockery, pans, empty milk bottles and remains of past meals littered the table. Cardboard boxes full of old copies of "Farmer's Weekly" and "Dairyman" were piled on two sagging armchairs. A tin bath reposed on the settee. He rummaged on top of the sideboard, among the debris of unopened correspondence, brica-brac and mouse droppings, and pulled out a clean hospital medicine box.

Within minutes, the injection had been given and various notes had been made in my diary regarding other services I would contact to provide help for Mr Hall in looking after his sister. I looked at my watch. Almost forty-five minutes had passed since I arrived, but with any luck I would soon be on my way. I was not to be let off so lightly. In the kitchen Farmer Hall was waiting for me.

"Ah've med ye a cuppa tea." His face beamed with the joy of my company. Guilt swept over me at my longing to dash away. He really was a fascinating and lovable character if only I had the time to enjoy him. Then I saw the tea. Greasy brown liquid swirled round in two dirty, chipped, white pint pots.

"Sit ye down and enjoy it," he said, pushing a pile of dirty washing off a wooden chair, his huge frame blocking my escape route.

I looked at his offering. A large dog hair floated on top next to another small piece of anonymous flotsam.

"I just want to see what ye think of me scar afore ye go."

God! – what was he going to show me? He pulled open his shirt to reveal a massive knotty scar just below his clavicle.

"What do ye think that was then?"

I hadn't the faintest idea but knew he would be far more pleased if he could 'baffle' me.

"Yer baffled aren't yer?" he cried in delight, "well I'll tell ye – it were one o'them caruncles! I 'ad five! – two on me back and one on each leg, – would ye like to see the other scars?"

"No – no!" I said quickly, "did you go to the doctor?"

"Naw!" he said scornfully, "ah told ye – I don't 'old wi' 'im – naw! – I treated meself!"

"What with?"

"Penicillin. I get it from t'vet for t' cows."

Again, I was horrified. "Mr Hall, you really mustn't treat yourself with other peoples' medication, and certainly not what you use for the cows!"

"Oh – ah know – ah know!" he was almost dancing with glee at the impression his story had made on me. "It said on t' syringe," he remembered the words with reverence, "for animals only!"

"You mean you injected yourself with a bovine dose? How did it affect you?"

"Well me caruncles got worse – coo! I were badly! – but that's the risk ye take when ye treat yerself. I asked me friend Sid Arcourt down t'road if he thought I ought to try it an I told him it said 'for animals only' and he said, "Well that should suit thee Seth, 'cos tha's just like a bloody gorilla, – tha's nowt to lose!"

"You could have killed yourself Mr Hall."

"Aye well ah'm still 'ere lass – now I mustn't keep ye – I'm sure yer busy. Ah shall watch out for ye next week, – I'm sure you'll enjoy another cuppa tea an a bit of a chat like."

As I drove away I wondered how many patients made free with each others pills? How many farmers like Mr Hall treated themselves with vetinary preparations? I remembered an item I had read in that mornings 'Yorkshire Post' – 'Farmer found dead in barn', said the headline. The coroner said there was no evidence to indicate the cause – it was a complete mystery. Perhaps I could give him some new ideas?

Ken and Sylvia were in their early fifties when I first visited. Sylvia had been diagnosed with a slowly growing tumour in her spine which was gradually paralysing her from the bottom up. Surgery had been attempted but was unsuccessful. It was academic whether the tumour was malignant or not – the result was the same.

By this time, Sylvia had been in hospital for a whole year and since nothing could be done, she was desperate just to go home. So Ken had given up his job to look after her. They had three children, grown up and gone, and three grandchildren.

I was asked to call to help and advise on nursing care and soon found that Ken, once taught, was quite capable of any nursing care Sylvia required, including changing her catheter. She was tiny and thin and at night Ken would carry her upstairs to bed. Soon it was only necessary to visit on a weekly supervisory basis. Theoretically this could have been a depressing call but it soon became the highlight of my week. In spite of being in pain most of the time, Sylvia was determined to remain cheerful.

Ken accepted the caring and the housework with an equally cheerful attitude. They were a perfect example of 'for better for worse' and making the best of things. They both had a marvellous sense of humour and after a short discussion about how things were I would enjoy a cup of coffee and some of Ken's baking while we shared funny anecdotes. At this stage Sylvia could still go out in the car with Ken lifting and strapping her in and putting the wheelchair in the boot, but gradually this became more difficult and they were trapped at home most of the time, especially in winter. Visitors became less frequent but Ken's brother Sam came faithfully every Monday afternoon and they appreciated his company. Occasionally Sam took his lady friend round to visit but this didn't work.

"She speaks to me as if I'm an imbecile," said an enraged Sylvia. "She bends down and raises her voice and says – 'are – you – in – pain?' then before I can answer she says to Ken, – 'ohh! Poor thing – is she in pain?'"

It was an unwritten rule that we did not become involved socially with patients but for them I broke it and often went round to supper, occasionally taking a friend as they enjoyed company so much. After my visit, Ken would walk me out to the car as this was our only opportunity to discuss any worries he had out of earshot of Sylvia.

"I want to know what's going to happen – what to expect when things get worse – you're the only one who will tell me anything. The doctor scuttles off as fast as he can if he senses an awkward question coming."

One day when Sylvia had had a few bad days and was obviously getting worse, Ken walked me out to the car. He was feeling down and for once he was thinking of himself as well.

"I've been wondering what on earth is going to happen to me when this is all over. Sylvia's had enough. I know what she's thinking but my life will be so empty. I don't know if I can get another job at my age and we've lost touch with so many friends." He was leaning on the garden gate. I put a hand on his arm.

"When this is over and when you're ready you're going to start a new life." He looked at me in amazement but I hoped he believed me.

Not long after that, Sylvia really started to deteriorate. The paralysis had crept up to the base of her lungs affecting her chest muscles and breathing was becoming more difficult. There was nothing to be done and I knew the next stage would be pneumonia, and a week later so it was. I took my lunch time sandwich and sat with them for a while. Sylvia just about knew I was there. Later on that night after I'd gone to bed Ken rang.

"Pam, I think she's gone"

"Do you want me to come?"

"No – there's nothing you can do. I've rung the children and they'll come."

I could only think I was glad Sylvia was out of pain at last.

A few months later I took Ken along to meet some friends. I was a member of a walking and social group in Leeds. They were very nice, interesting people and I knew they'd welcome Ken as he could be relied upon to be an asset in any company. He thoroughly enjoyed the walk and joined the group and I could see he was beginning to look forward again. A short time later, a bright attractive lady a few years younger than Ken, joined us. She had been widowed two years previously. She and Ken hit it off like a house on fire and they married two years later. We are still great friends.

* * *

It was a lovely bright sunny day and I called a cheery good morning to George the milkman as I went down the path to my third visit of the day. Mrs Harrison was in the kitchen with Dr Archie Craig. Mr Harrison had suddenly worsened the previous week and had been taken to hospital where he died. I had called to collect some nursing equipment just as Mrs Harrison was showing Archie the death certificate from the hospital.

"He wasn't suffering from what you said he'd got Doctor, it says something different here."

I dug Archie in the ribs and said "wrong again!" His usual sense of humour was missing on this occasion. Without looking at me he said, "The nurse is very busy this morning. We shall not detain her." Pompous so and so I thought, but I grabbed my sheets and bed pan and hurried off.

Outside I found the milkman waiting for me, looking anxious. Finding the milk at one of his customers hadn't been taken in for two days he had ventured inside and found an old man in his bed.

"He looks very poorly – I shouldn't be surprised if he's dead – will you have a look at him?"

The front door of the upstairs council flat was open and I found George's old man just as he'd said. He was in a moribund condition but was still alive, just. George had come in behind me. "What do you think?" he asked.

"I think we need to get him into hospital… has he any family?"

"Don't know – he lives alone – don't know much about him," said George.

"Okay – I'll ask his downstairs neighbour if she knows who his doctor is."

After banging on the door of the bottom flat for what seemed an age a bad tempered young woman appeared in her nightie, with a snotty nosed toddler clinging to her legs, and demanded to know why I'd knocked her up at this effing time. It was ten o'clock. No she didn't know who his doctor was and she didn't effing care. I decided not to ask if I could use her phone and went back to Mrs Harrison's and sent for an ambulance. I carried on and forgot about it.

Two days later Miss Burton asked me to come to her office.

"Ah! – Sister Baines – I've had a complaint about you." She looked at me coldly.

My heart sank but I said nothing, merely returning her gaze. "From a Dr. Gordon from Hadleigh." I was mystified.

"What about?"

"Evidently you sent a patient of his into hospital without consulting him."

"How could I consult him? – I didn't know who the patient's doctor was. The patient was unconscious, verging on death, what was I supposed to do?"

"Yes, well, I don't want to hear any more complaints about you."

I was furious. This was so unfair. I stood my ground.

"Tell me Miss Burton what should I have done? What would you have done?"

Of course she couldn't answer and at that moment the phone rang – saved by the bell!

I made my way out of the building wondering if this petty critical style of nurse management would ever change. We had put up with it as student nurses but nothing altered when we became qualified, and we were given no credit for the good work we did, and constantly told off as if we were naughty children, at every opportunity. I wondered if senior management had any idea how many good nurses they lost due to petty tyrant nurse managers.

* * *

As I looked at the divide in the lane I cursed myself for not transferring the instructions from the message pad to my work diary. Was it right or left? Some vague memory told me it was right but the lane to the left looked a better made road. Left it would be!

I set off with my wheels running on ancient flagstones, worn down with centuries of use, only just wide enough for a car. There was a high bank on the left topped by a thick hedge. On the right was another hedge which to my discomfort soon disappeared to reveal a sheer thirty foot drop into a wood with a stream at the bottom.

I rattled on and on, round left hand bends and right hand bends and as the path suddenly steepened I glimpsed a Victorian house at the bottom of the hill. I had a strong feeling this was not Brockett Hall Farm. The house almost clung to the hillside with a small garden back and front, and very little flat land on which to turn my car.

As I walked up the path the front door opened and a shabbily dressed, bad tempered looking man stood there.

"Good morning – is this Brockett Hall Farm?" I asked hesitantly, withering under his scowl.

"No its not and this is private property – didn't you see the sign at the top of the lane?"

"Er – no – I'm sorry. Could you possibly move your car so I can turn round?"

"No, certainly not." His eyes glittered with anger, "you shouldn't have come down here."

124

He turned and started to close the door. Panic seized me; I could not reverse back up that awful track!

"Please – it will only take you a minute – I can't reverse up that dangerous track!" The door was closed in my face.

I did reverse back up the track, stopping and straightening up again and again, with one eye on the sheer drop. It must have taken nearly half an hour and when I arrived safely at the top my arms and legs were shaking and my neck and head ached with the beginning of a migraine. I sat with my head resting on the steering wheel feeling sweat running down my back. Never, never would I go back down that track. It was to be hoped the unpleasant creature who lived in the wood, and any family he may have, would stay in perfect health because if they needed a district nurse it was not going to be me.

Finally collecting myself I turned on to the right hand track where I should have been in the first place. Halfway along to the farm, which soon came into view, was a sharp right turn and suddenly I had to stand on my brakes as a collie shot out from the hedge and into my path. He ran in circles in front of my bonnet then disappeared just as suddenly.

I crept gingerly forward and just as my nerves were settling down he leapt out again. I realised that this was how he got his kicks and probably there was no danger he would be hit; he knew what he was doing. Pulling up in the farm yard I noticed him hiding in the hedge waiting for my return journey.

The farm house had the usual neglected air to be expected where father and son lived together, with no woman's touch. My message said 'Mr Hudson, 78 years, leg ulcers.'

The path to the front door was impassable with overgrown bushes, an old pram and the remains of an ancient cooker lying on its side. I headed round the back and picked my way through some hens and a couple of ducks, trying to avoid piles of their excreta.

The back door was partly open as it rested askew on one hinge. I tried to find a clean patch on which to knock, as it was covered with a mixture of mud and manure. A voice shouted 'Come in,' and I made my way down a gloomy passage, with damp wallpaper hanging off in places. Following the light and sounds it led me into a large kitchen cum living room which boasted a huge range with an open fire. It had large pipes leading from it round the room and through the ceiling. I assumed it was a Heath Robinson type of central heating.

"Who are you then? Come nearer – lets 'ave a look at you!" The old man sat in an ancient wooden rocking chair, pulled right up to the range.

I introduced myself and told him Dr. Smith had asked me to attend to his sore legs.

"Has he now? Well that's okay, to me – they're certainly giving me some gyp."

He seemed delighted to see me which was half the battle. He had been wrapping his legs in a motley assortment of rags and it was a miracle they weren't too badly infected. I dressed them with my sterile supplies and firm bandages and asked him not to touch them until my next visit.

"Ee lass that's grand – better already. I'll not touch them, don't you worry!"

I told him I would visit three times a week until his legs had healed, and checked he was taking his antibiotics properly. I had just settled at the table to fill in his paper work, which was left in the house so my colleagues could follow treatment instructions on my day off, when a terrible ear splitting rattling noise started, emanating from the range, and everything in the room started to shake. Accompanied by the hissing and rumbling sounds of water boiling, I watched in awe as all the pipes of the 'central heating' banged and shook. A cup and saucer danced towards me across the table and I caught it as it shot off the edge. A pan fell off a shelf above Mr Hudson's head and he caught it with one hand, without batting an eye-lid.

"How do you like me central heating?" Mr Hudson shouted above the din, an unmistakeable air of pride in his voice.

"It looks dangerous to me." I shouted back, feeling glad I was ready to go.

"I put it in meself in 1924," he said proudly, "it's nivver let us down!" I headed for the door. Mr Hudson tried to explain that 'Ermintrude' would probably jump out at me. I told him we'd already met and I'd see him on Wednesday. He said he'd look forward to it.

As the weeks went by I realised why he was so pleased to have a nurse visiting, apart from the improvement in his ulcers. His son Graham had never married and Mr Hudson would have dearly loved to have a woman about the place again, since his wife had died ten years ago.

"He's nivver got off the ground in that department," he confided to me, "too slow to catch a cold."

I met Graham once or twice as I visited the farm. He was reasonably presentable, if somewhat shy and awkward.

"Couldn't you fancy him lass? – you'd suit us reet well!" I told him I was otherwise engaged which somewhat dashed his hopes.

"The last time there was any romance in the air, shall we say, was a post lady a while back. He took her t' pictures one night but then she got moved to another area and that was last 'o that – too slow to catch a cold." I left him shaking his head and staring into the fire. Graham waved to me from his tractor as I drove down the lane. I sent a silent prayer up that one day he'd find someone. She'd probably cope with his father but I wasn't sure about that central heating.

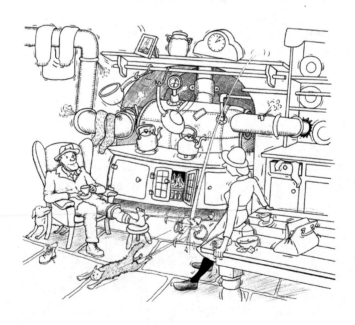

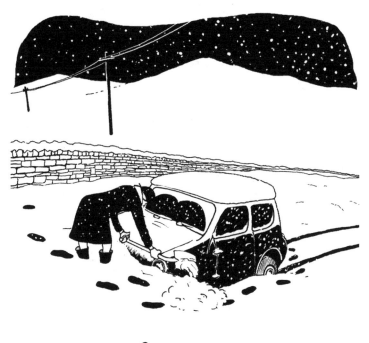

Chapter 8

"Have you seen this?" Jennifer marched into the office and threw the local paper on to my desk.

"What?" Margaret and I chorused together.

"The front page! The headlines!"

We were having one of the worst spells of snow and freezing conditions we had ever endured. The chairman of the Health Authority had been interviewed about how staff were managing to get to work to keep the hospitals running. The whole article gushed with praise for the hospital nurses whose endeavours evidently compared with climbing the Matterhorn by breakfast and Everest before tea. The district nurses weren't mentioned, when in fact every visit we made was a triumph over adversity.

Most of us had been lucky; several times when we'd been stuck, people had appeared from nowhere, like guardian angels, to give us a push. Sally from the Bridgend lot had skidded in her brand new car into a wall, and a rumour reached us that some determined soul had managed to reach a farm in the wilds of Hebden Bridge only to have to stay the night as she was trapped by blizzard conditions. The council workers did a heroic job trying to keep the main roads clear but on all the minor roads off the beaten track the snow was level with the wall tops. We weighted our boots down and carried spades and sacks to put under the wheels.

An occasional parking space at the roadside had been dug out, and often when nurse and doctor arrived at the same time there was an undignified scramble for the precious patch. Sheila from Bridgend had the bright idea of filling our car boots with sacks of potatoes to provide ballast, which we could then eat. When the thaw came, most of us found our potatoes had gone rotten. We tried to keep to the main roads, walking the rest and leaving our cars on the main road overnight. Sally drove round in her spare car, an almost vintage Morris Minor which was surprisingly good at going up un-gritted hills.

"I saw you all sitting crying in your fancy cars at the bottom of the hill, while I sailed up no bother!" she said frequently.

Margaret had an old lady in the wilds who was overdue for a vitamin B injection and although we kept telling her she wasn't about to die for lack of it,

Margaret set off with a spade, like Captain Scott, in a valiant attempt to reach her patient. She walked along the dry stone wall top until she could see the house, and then tried gingerly to test the frozen snow in the lane. Surprisingly it held her weight until with the next step she disappeared from sight, leaving her hat on top of the snow. She had been walking on top of abandoned cars.

The doctors at my surgery decided we'd have a competition to see who had the most hair-raising experience. It was no contest when Dr Galbraith junior skidded at the top of an enormous 1 in 4 hill and ended up with his back end hanging over a low wall, and his hair standing on end. The worst of it was over when I had my nastiest shock.

It had been at least three days since the last snowfall, usually ample time for our gritters to make the most dangerous roads safe. However, I was still doubtful about my regular shortcut down a steep cobbled hill which shortened my journey to one of the villages by five minutes or so. Then the car in front of me turned right to go down the lane – perhaps he knew something I didn't. I followed and realised our mistake at the top of the hill. It was like the Cresta run and too late to turn back, my car took off in an uncontrollable slide.

Halfway down the hill the car in front slid sideways, then, gathering speed hit the wall at the bottom with a sickening crunch: with my heart in my mouth, and with my hands and knees shaking, I watched a group of children making their way up the hill, laughing and slipping and hanging on to the rail; there was absolutely no hope I could stop. Gently touching my brakes the car veered to the left and oh! – joy of joys! – the front wheels caught tenuously on some ashes someone had put out. My car stopped. Gingerly hanging on to the bonnet I managed to move to some less icy ground. Then, to my horror another car was sliding down from the top. I waited helplessly for it to crash into mine but as the white faced occupant neared he suddenly shot to the right over a low wall and disappeared down a steep field.

I knocked at the door of the house where my guardian angel had thrown out the ashes. A quick phone call to the Highways department and all I had to do was wait for rescue and hope no more cars would come down the hill. Sure enough, about fifteen minutes later, a lorry started reversing up the hill towards me. On the back, in amongst the sand and salt, stood a little bandy legged old man wielding a shovel. As he threw out the grit the lorry reversed up. Drawing level with me he gave me a look of pure disgust.

"Nobody in their right mind would've come down here on a day like this," he said, throwing a shovelfull on my shoes.

"It's been here three days. I thought you would have made it safe by now." I retorted as I rolled off carefully on my way.

Two weeks later it was still snowing on and off. Our wonderful council workers kept the roads gritted, particularly the hills – and we had plenty of those. Every night we went to bed anxious as to what we would find next morning, and most of us had broken nights, getting up to peep out warily several times. Just when we thought it was over, back came the snow with a vengeance.

That night almost the whole of West Yorkshire gridlocked. Although it had been forecast, the blizzard started several hours earlier than anticipated. The gritters set off too late and became stuck in the home going – or not going – rush hour traffic.

I was a long way from home as I left my last visit. It was dark and as I headed towards the main road, I couldn't believe how thick the snow had become in such a short time, and glancing up, could see plenty more where that had come from.

A short but very steep hill lay between me and the by-pass and knowing I daren't slow down, or stop at the top, I blew my horn and flashed my lights as I shot out on to the road, thankfully not under the wheels of a lorry. The traffic soon became bumper to bumper but at least it was still moving slowly, until, almost at my turn off we all ground to a halt and sat watching the snow gleaming like flakes of crystal in the mass of headlights of four lanes of traffic. An hour later, inching slowly forward, I managed to turn off the by-pass and slithering down to the main road at the bottom, I spotted a small vacant patch where I could abandon my car.

On every road I could see traffic queued, headlights glaring, engines running, going nowhere. I knew I had about five miles to walk to get home but I was so grateful I had got as far as I had. I had an umbrella, there was no icy wind blowing, and I was wearing my comfy flat duty shoes. I could reach home and a warm bed that night which was more than most occupants of the cars could hope for.

Five minutes later, I staggered into a pub to have a quick drink and buy some crisps and peanuts to fortify myself. It was packed with people and a kind of blitz spirit was evident as stories of skids, bumps and cars abandoned were shared and passed round. Most of them seemed settled in for the night in the warmth.

"You're not going back out there are you Nurse? – come and join us!" shouted one chap as I waved and headed for the door.

I decided to walk down the middle of the road as the snow on the pavements was so thick; and every so often, to my amazement a woman would jump out of her car and ask if she could join me. I can only imagine seeing my uniform meant someone safe and sensible. My answer was, "as long as you can keep up!" as most of these women were unsuitably dressed and wearing high heels and as far as I was concerned tonight was every man for himself.

At one stage there were ten of us, arousing frequent wolf whistles from the men in the cars. Two of my ladies were crying because they were lost and their boyfriends would be worrying about them. My reply that their boyfriends were probably also lost and only worrying about themselves didn't go down too well but by striding along on my lovely flat shoes I eventually left them behind. It was almost midnight when I reached home and had to be up early next morning to walk back and dig my car out.

* * *

North Green was the prettiest of my villages, on the boundary with Bradford. On a warm sunny day it was a joy to drive round. On this particular day it was hot and sunny and anything but a joy, as I pulled on my furry winter boots.

I strode up the path to Mr and Mrs Clark's cottage on the main street. Mr Clark had suffered a stroke a few weeks ago and could have been cared for at home, providing his wife was capable of looking after him, with my help. Mrs Clark was most certainly not capable of looking after him however, as she seemed to me to have more problems than her husband – mental health problems; in fact she seemed to be going completely round the bend.

She wasn't feeding her husband or giving him anything to drink in between my visits and I couldn't seem to get this through to her G.P. Dr. Goldie's surgery was over the border in Bradford area so he was what we called an out-side G.P. He was a blunt Yorkshire man not given to visiting his patients unless it was a matter of life and death.

"What's up with you woman! I visited last week, they were alright then," he exclaimed when I called him.

"But she's not feeding him Dr Goldie, he's neglected and she can't cope. She's in a world of her own."

"Aye – well – I'll pop in again next week."

Don't bother, I thought, he'll be dead by then.

The worst aspect of the problem for me was that she wasn't feeding the dog either. It was a Sheltie, a small Collie, called Hedley and what had been a rather bad tempered creature was driven by hunger into being a vicious man-eater, or at least 'nurse-eater', hence the boots to save my ankles.

"Mrs Clark – hello! – it's the nurse!"

I knocked at the door and peered through the letter box. I could see Mrs Clark sitting in a dream stroking Hedley who, hearing me, hurled himself at the letter box, snarling and yapping hysterically.

"Put the dog in the kitchen please Mrs Clark, – no – don't open the door yet – put – the – dog – in – the – kitchen." I watched her dreamily weaving towards the kitchen with Hedley jumping up eagerly round her hoping she might put some food in his bowl. As she opened the door I saw too late that the back door was wide open. Two seconds later Hedley flew round the side of the building and hurled himself at me. Snarling with a mixture of joy and fury he sank his teeth into my boots. This caused less damage than without the boots but it still wasn't pleasant and I was glad to be driving away half an hour later, having attended to Mr. Clark and found something in the larder to feed them both and an ungrateful Hedley, who didn't seem to get it that I was all that stood between him and starvation.

A few days later Dr Goldie rang me.

"You might have told me about the damn dog! – bit a great lump out of me and tore my trousers!"

"Really? – what a shame." I replied.

"Well, anyway, I've sent them both in – he's in the General and she's in the Psychiatric unit – oh and the dog's gone to the R.S.P.C.A."

Good old Hedley!

* * *

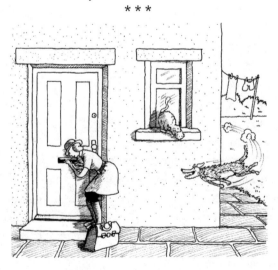

"I was better looked after when I was in the jungle in Burma surrounded by the Japs."

Brian had been ill for about two years and for some reason it had taken a long time to get a diagnosis. He was suffering from a deficiency of vitamin B12, which was a reasonably common condition but he felt his G.P. had been slow on the uptake and he should have had blood tests done a lot sooner. He also suffered from recurrent depression due to having been a prisoner of war in the hands of the Japanese. Brian felt his G.P. had put all his symptoms down to his depression and had failed to look further.

"During the war the army doctors were marvellous. We had the best treatment available in double quick time – until we were captured of course."

Brian fell silent, going in his mind to a dark place full of unimaginable horrors. I didn't ask as I knew he didn't want to talk about it. He had once said to me, "Do you wonder I get depressed when I've seen things no one should have to see? – two of my best mates beheaded in front of me."

The wonderful thing about Brian was that he had managed somehow to keep his sense of humour. A lot of the time visiting him was a delight.

"Now then Mistress Niven – what have you come for?" he would tease.

At the time, a popular programme on television was 'Dr. Finlay's Casebook,' and Mistress Niven was an unqualified district nurse – a very large middle aged busybody of a character. His greeting never failed to make me laugh.

The treatment for his B12 deficiency was an injection every three months and it was lovely to see him feeling better. Things seemed to be looking up but then he suffered two set backs in his life.

He lived in a small cottage with his mother. He hadn't been able to cope with marriage after the war. Unfortunately the Council decided to demolish the small row of cottages to widen the road. Brian and his mother were to be given a Council flat. They were devastated and the worry of it caused Brian to sink into depression again, and his mother also became ill. Just before they were due to move into the flat she had a stroke and died. Brian was distraught – his life was collapsing round him. He moved into the flat but he was struggling to cope. Before long he had to be admitted to a psychiatric hospital yet again. When he felt a bit better he wrote to me.

"I'm in really good company here. There are two hospital consultants, an M.P., and several clergymen! I wonder who are mad? – us? – or you lot outside!" Sadly a few months later in spite of observation, he found a way to commit suicide. His long journey from Burma was over.

* * *

It was not going to be an easy visit.

"Mrs Sugden's an awkward, uncooperative old devil," my colleague had warned me.

"And what's more, she has this budgie flying round the room doing whoopsies all over the place. It landed on my hat yesterday, right in the middle of giving her injection – I got such a shock it would have served her right if I'd broken the needle!"

"Perhaps the budgie is all she has in the world to give affection to," I suggested in mitigation of Mrs. Sugden's dreadful sins.

"Right! But she should keep it locked up in it's cage. She lets it do what it likes and it rules the household, terrorising anyone who dares to step over the threshold – no wonder the neighbours have stopped going in to help her – and it's so unhygienic anyway!" she continued, "still you shouldn't have any problems tomorrow on my day off."

"Why not?"

"Oh! I told her you wouldn't put up with it. You'll have to shut that budgie up when Sister Baines comes, I said, she hates budgies."

"Thanks very much – she's going to love me!"

This was typical of my colleague. She suffered from a Nightingale complex – a desperate desire to be seen as a ministering angel and every time a patient had to be told off she would use me as the ogre, the ultimate threat.

"You'll have to get the bed downstairs by weekend," she would tell the relatives, "Sister Baines will refuse to bring the patient down these dangerous stairs!" or "Sister Baines won't let you smoke in bed, like I do, Mr Crowther – you'll have to stop it," to some poor old man whose last remaining pleasure in life was his pipe. Since the response elicited by this kind of remark was usually, "She can mind her own business then can't she?" not much was achieved by this approach except to undermine the patients' confidence in me and put Sister Green definitely one up.

So it was with some apprehension that I walked up Mrs. Sugden's path and let myself in at the front door. A cupboard like hall led straight into the living room where

Mrs Sugden sat upright in a large old-fashioned wooden bed in the far corner. Since her illness, her world had shrunk to this one room where she lived, ate and slept.

"Good morning, Mrs. Sugden!" I said brightly, "I'm Sister Baines. I'm sure Sister Green told you I was coming to see you today."

"Oh aye! – she told me alright." She glowered at me from the bed.

It was not a good start but no worse than I had expected, and at least I had not yet been bombed by the bowel opening budgie. I glanced warily round the room and then I saw him in his cage by the window. He sat silently on his perch, watching me with the same menacing expression as his owner.

"You've no need to worry, I've shut him up like I was told," she cried sharply, "and he's right miserable I can tell you. Fancy being frightened of a budgie!"

I decided to ignore this as although not enjoying being cast in the role of villain by my so-called friend and colleague, I had to agree with her about the problem of hygiene and I was rather nervous of birds flying round my head – in fact I had never liked budgies, feeling sorry for them if they were imprisoned in cages, and for myself if they were not.

I busied myself making my patient's bed.

"How are you feeling this morning?"

"Considering there's nowt wrong with me – alright."

She was too proud to admit her frailty, born of a generation used to long hours of toil at the loom, unable in those days to afford to be ill.

"You've had pneumonia you know." I pointed out gently.

"Rubbish! It were no'but a heavy cold, but my bum's like a pin cushion with all those needles you lot have stuck in me!"

I felt it would be useless to point out that the anti-biotics had saved her life and that it would only provoke further argument.

"Well, cheer up, last one today, then I'll help you to have a wash."

"That's what I need, a nice wash, with plenty of hot water – you'd better put the kettle on hadn't you?" she said with a strange smile on her face.

The budgie wasn't smiling as I passed him on my way to the kitchen. He was swinging slightly on his perch, feathers tucked tightly in all round him, in sulky fashion, still reproachfully watching me.

The cooker was a solid, pre-war, gas monstrosity, on legs with feet that had clawed holes in the lino. It looked as awkward and un-cooperative as Mrs Sugden and the budgie put together. I had engaged in battle with this type of appliance in many an old kitchen and knew it's tricks of old. They were difficult to light and just as you had almost given up hope and bent your face over the burner to see what was wrong, it would ignite in an attempt to denude your face of eyebrows and eyelashes. I looked on the shelf above the cooker for the matches. There were none there, nor were they in any of the other obvious places.

"I can't find the matches Mrs. Sugden," I called to the old lady.

"No – they're not in there." I heard her reply.

I returned to the room. "Where are they then?"

She looked at me silently, savouring her moment, then, triumphantly, she could resist no longer.

"They're in t'budgie's cage!"

* * *

I was having a strange morning. Visiting a new patient at Southfield whose home was a small holding up a very narrow track, I found I had nowhere to park except on a rather small patch of ground which had a goat tethered on it. Neither I, nor the goat, was very pleased about me leaving my car on its territory.

The house was dark and gloomy, surrounded by trees, all swaying madly in the wind. After a lot of knocking I heard the sound of keys turning in locks and bolts being drawn, accompanied by a lot of cursing and muttering. Finally the door opened to reveal a grim faced man with dark glittering eyes and long unkempt hair. He stared at me, waiting for me to speak.

"Good morning. I'm the district nurse and I've come to see a Mr Jakovski."

He glared at me, then stood back and silently extended a bony finger in the direction of a corridor to the right. Trying not to shudder I followed the passage and found Mr Jakovski in bed in a small cluttered room. He had scalded both legs below the knee and as I removed the rags they were wrapped in I didn't like the look of them at all. Mr Jakovski's G.P. had told me he was Polish and that his command of English was poor, and as I tried to chat to him it was obvious he didn't understand. He also seemed to be in the land of the bewildered.

As I finished his bandages and pulled the bed clothes back over him he suddenly sat up and gripped my arm, pushing his face near to mine in an alarming manner.

"You must save yourself, my dear, the Bolsheviks are coming! Save yourself! hurry! – hurry!"

Startled I hurried in search of the other weirdo who'd let me in. Popping my head round a door I found him, and opened my mouth to tell him I would visit again tomorrow and that I thought the doctor ought to see Mr Jakovski's legs, but the vision that met my eyes stunned me to silence. The room was full of witches! Two doll sized models of witches on broomsticks sat atop the dresser. Their faces were ugly and menacing. Small witches dangled from several places on the ceiling. A stags head peered at me from above the fireplace. Little black witches complete with hats and broomsticks hung from every branch of its antlers.

As I was gazing at this unbelievable sight my eye was caught by a very amateurish oil painting to the right of the stag's head. In the background was a house, dark and forbidding, almost hidden in trees with menacing branches, and in the foreground stood a woman with long black hair, wearing a black cloak. Her expression was pure evil. On the other side of the stag's head was a large photograph of Hitler!

The nameless man spoke at last.

"I see you are admiring the painting of my wife."

"I'll –er- see you –er- again tomorrow." I stuttered and shot out of the front door. With a quick look round to see if there were any Bolsheviks about I headed for my car. As I leant into the back to put my briefcase away I felt a sharp tug on my mackintosh. Damn! It was the goat!

I tried to kick backwards but it hung on for dear life and as I struggled to get out of my mac there was a loud ripping sound and I caught sight of a piece of blue material disappearing between the goat's teeth. What a nightmare of a visit and I had to repeat it all tomorrow!

Glancing at my watch I saw I was almost late for a meeting with a social worker. Mr and Mrs Field were totally incapable of looking after themselves and needed to go into care. They were both suffering from dementia and were doubly incontinent at times, usually as they were perambulating about the house. Several home helps had left or refused to visit again. Beds in the geriatric wards or care homes were in short supply but if the home helps wouldn't visit, and there were no relatives, something had to be done.

Two days previously Mrs. Field had been found wandering down the road dressed only in a vest and a pair of Mr. Field's hobnailed boots. In desperation I had asked social services to send a social worker to meet me at the house to see for themselves.

There was no social worker to be seen as I pulled up outside the house. A young man in a long overcoat and fingerless gloves was leaning against the wall rolling up a cigarette with tobacco from a tin. His hair hung in long plaits, Rastafarian style. I got out of the car wondering if the social worker was already inside.

"Oh hi man! You must be the district nurse," the young man grinned at me.

"Good grief! Don't tell me you're the social worker!" I said, then realised how rude it sounded.

"Yeah well – times are changing – identify with the client group and all that." He seemed to have taken no offence, but I couldn't see how he was identifying with an old couple in their eighties.

Mr and Mrs Field were sitting in their living room – up and dressed, albeit in a strange selection of garments. She seemed to be wearing some of his clothes and he was definitely wearing some of hers.

"They don't look too bad at all" said my juvenile social worker cheerfully.

"Don't start that!" I cried, "you've no idea." I asked them when they had last eaten. They looked vague and Mr. Field said he was hungry. In the kitchen there was a smell of gas and an unlit gas ring was on. I suggested we had a look upstairs.

"You go first." I gave the young man a bit of a push. He looked at me with suspicion but set off up the narrow, dark staircase, then suddenly stopped.

"Ooh! I think I've trodden in something awful!" His face turned a pale shade of green and he dashed outside.

"I hope you take my point." I said as I found him trying to clean up on some grass, still pale. Two days later a place was found in a care home for the Fields. I was so pleased as it was nearly Christmas and I'd hated to think of them struggling on their own.

Driving home for lunch through the council estate I stopped to give Mrs. Achroyd her vitamin B12 injection for pernicious anaemia. She had decorated her Christmas tree and sprayed 'Merry Christmas to one and all' in her front window. The Grundys opposite had sprayed their window in competition. 'Naff off to one and all at Christmas' it proclaimed.

Chapter 9

I stood on the doorstep and waited for someone to answer my knock. The November afternoon was damp and gloomy and I shivered as I glanced at the neglected house next door, surrounded by the overgrown foliage of a garden which had returned to nature.

The door opened and a middle aged woman stood in front of me. I could smell home baked bread and feel warmth drifting from the kitchen to the hall. The contrast with the house next door was complete.

"Ah! – it's Mrs Pickles isn't it?" I tried to charm the somewhat stony faced woman with a bright smile. "I'm sorry to bother you but I can't get in next door at Mrs Walmsley's and I wondered if you'd seen an ambulance: we've been trying to get her into hospital you see, and she may have already gone?"

"Oh yes, she's gone alright; the ambulance came about an hour ago and not before time in my view, she's not fit to be living on her own, in that house, wandering about at all hours of the night; you wouldn't think we had a health service; I don't know what we pay all those stamps for –"

"Oh I'm glad you saw the ambulance," I cut in, thinking 'not that you miss much.'

"Well, I just hope she doesn't come back this time, they should never have let her come home last time she was in. It's a worry living next door to a house like that, it lowers the tone of the whole neighbourhood and........."

"Well, you see, we can't make her stay in hospital, Mrs Pickles," I cut in again, "she refuses to be admitted most of the time and when we do manage to persuade her she takes her own discharge as soon as she feels a bit better."

I smiled at Mrs Pickles again, to no avail. To Mrs Pickles I was one of 'them', part of a Health Service which ought to be able to solve all problems by the wave of a magic wand.

"Well I don't know about that but she's been going funny in the head for a long time now and it's time she was kept in hospital and someone had a good look through that house," – she pointed to the house next door, "because it's not her I'm worried about, it's **him!**"

"Him? Do you mean Mr Walmsley?"

"Yes I do."

"Mr Walmsley died two years ago Mrs Pickles; surely you knew?"

"Of course I knew! But where is he? That's what I want to know, because a coffin went in but no coffin came out and if you ask me, he's still in there!"

Mrs Pickles had dropped her bombshell and now stood with arms folded, her mouth in a straight line, watching me.

"But there must have been a funeral Mrs Pickles, perhaps you've missed seeing them leave the house that's all?"

"Listen!" Mrs Pickles addressed me impatiently. "I didn't know he'd died until I saw the coffin being delivered, they'd kept themselves to themselves that much. Anyway, I went round to offer my sympathy and enquire about the funeral. She said she hadn't made all the arrangements and more or less tried to shut the door in my face – just fancy! So I asked her to let me know when she had but I heard nothing from her, so I watched the house; well the weather was fine and I was gardening, but a whole week went by and no-one came out of that house, dead or alive! I'm telling you, he's still in there!"

"There has to be some explanation, perhaps there was no funeral, perhaps his body was donated for medical research."

"It's still got to come out of the house hasn't it? – and I know it didn't. Anyway, she said he'd been buried at St Mary's."

"There you are then"

"Unfortunately the vicar doesn't agree," said Mrs Pickles triumphantly.

"Do you mean you've discussed this with the vicar?"

"Well, after a week passed with no sign of a funeral, I went round to see Mrs Walmsley. She didn't want to open the door but after I'd banged and banged she opened it just a crack – on the chain. I asked her when the funeral was to be and she said it had been the previous day. I asked what time it had been and she got very flustered."

I felt sorry for Mrs Walmsley as I looked at the intimidating Mrs Pickles. It must have felt like being interrogated by the Gestapo.

"I asked where he was buried and she said 'St Mary's' and just shut the door."

"What did you say about the vicar?"

"Oh – well, I went round the graveyard looking for a newly dug grave and there wasn't one so I went to see the vicar. He'd never heard of the Walmsleys."

"Perhaps she was confused. She must have been upset. Perhaps she meant St Michael's."

"No! I went there as well. He isn't buried in any graveyard round here." She bent her face near to mine and hissed through her teeth, "He's still in there!"

"I've been visiting Mrs Walmsley for the past twelve months and I haven't seen a coffin – where do you think it is?"

The reply came instantaneously. "In that library cum study – where he always sat when he was alive."

Suddenly I remembered my first visit to Mrs Walmsley. I had gone automatically to the room where Mr Walmsley had always been when I attended him.

"Not in there!" Mrs Walmsley had called from the hall, in an agitated manner and as my hand had turned the handle, I realised it was locked. It seemed odd at the time – now it seemed sinister.

"Have you told anyone else about this Mrs Pickles?"

"Only the vicar of St Mary's. I told him the whole story and that it ought to be investigated but he didn't take much notice. He said he couldn't possibly interfere and he was quite sure there was some explanation. So I said if he wouldn't do anything I'd have to go to the Police and he said I ought to think most carefully before taking such a step. Well, it's alright for him isn't it? His neighbours probably don't keep dead bodies behind locked doors…"

"And did you?" I chipped in sharply.

"Did I what?"

"Go to the Police?"

"Well, I wanted to, I felt it was my public duty, but my husband said we ought not to get involved. Anyway, I knew the truth would have to come out sooner or later as it wouldn't be long before she died or had to be taken away."

I was struck by Mrs Pickles' lack of any sign of compassion for her neighbour. The woman almost revelled in poor Mrs. Walmsley's demise.

"So I'm glad to tell you about this because now, the authorities will have to do something. The sooner you have a jolly good look round next door, the better! There's a key at Mrs Simpson's, at number 42, we could go together." Mrs Pickles was positively eager now.

"But Mrs. Pickles, we can't possibly go into Mrs. Walmsley's house without her permission and we have no grounds for doing such a thing, it's out of the question."

"Do you mean you're going to do nothing? – after all I've told you."

"I shall mention your anxiety about the whereabouts of Mr Walmsley's remains to Dr Smith." I said pompously.

"Oh! – and a fat lot he'll do about it knowing him," snapped Mrs. Pickles. I started to back away down the path.

"Thank you for letting me know about the ambulance."

"Just you see that something gets done," she shouted at my retreating back, "it's a disgrace, all those stamps we pay and what do we get for it?"

I could still hear her voice through the gloom, it was almost dark now. I climbed wearily into my car mulling over the conversation. I looked again at the dark neglected house and my mind drifted back to the first time I had been asked to visit.

Mr Walmsley had been the first to require the attention of the nursing service. I had thought the house was uninhabited at first. The windows were dark and dirty with yellowed lace curtains hanging in holes. The paint was brown and peeling off the rotting frames. I checked my diary entry: Mr Walmsley, 32 Cedar Drive, dressing to leg ulcers. This was it. The gate refused to move at first, then as I heaved my bag against it, it swung inward off it's hinges. I forced my way up the path as briars snagged my black tights and over hanging bushes caught at my hair. It had been raining and water dripped down my face from the heavy leaves. I knocked on the glass panel of the heavy door and tried the handle, locked of course. I knocked again and as I stood waiting, listening, rain from broken guttering dripped onto my hat and down my neck. Eventually, after banging a third time, I heard a shuffling noise in the hall.

"Who is it?"

"It's the district nurse, Mrs Walmsley, Dr. Smith asked me to call"

There was a long pause.

"What for?"

"I've come to attend to your husband's leg." Heavens above! She must know!

Another pause, then a lot of muttering followed by the rattling of keys, bolts and chains being unfastened by clumsy age-worn fingers.

The door opened just enough for the old lady to size up her visitor.

"You'd better come in then," she said, sounding as if she was doing me a favour. I stepped into a cold dark hall crammed with furniture. The old lady was dressed in a long tweed overcoat, torn in several places and of a style long gone. A faded brown beret hid her hair except for a few wild straggles. She was wearing fingerless woolly gloves and below her wrinkled stockings was a pair of down-at-heel leather boots. She shambled off down a corridor and I looked about me as I followed.

The wallpaper was faded and dirty and looked as if it had been there at least forty years. Several hideous ornaments and statuettes were covered in cobwebs. 'The Boyhood of Raleigh' hung from a picture rail at the foot of the staircase, next to a huge mahogany grandfather clock, long since stopped. The old woman showed me into a room at the end of the passage.

"There's a nurse here Hector, come to attend to your bad leg." Then she was gone, leaving me with my patient. The curtains were drawn and at first I could hardly see him, the room was so dark. He was sitting in a wing armchair next to an open coal fire, dressed in pyjama bottoms and a black quilted smoking jacket, with a small round black satin hat to match.

"Good morning Mr. Walmsley," I ventured. He looked at me curiously.

"Who are you?" Not again!

Once I had explained, he reluctantly allowed me to dress his leg and even admitted grudgingly that it felt better.

I had to attend for the next few months and slowly I developed a relationship of trust with the old couple. Unfortunately, I was unable to persuade them to allow anyone else into the house to help them. I was sorry when Mr Walmsley had a heart attack and died and it was not long after that that Mrs Walmsley needed attention. That was the day I remembered her becoming agitated as I tried the door of the library and found it locked.

That night I slept badly. I kept dreaming about coffins lying in book lined rooms. I mentioned Mrs. Pickles' suspicions to Dr Smith the next morning.

"Well what do you want me to do about it?" he snapped.

"Well – I don't know really – what can we do?"

"Precisely!" So, that for the time being, was that.

A few months later I was passing 32 Cedar Drive, Mrs. Walmsley had died in hospital and had never returned to the house. Outside stood a large house clearance van. A rather rough looking character was pushing boxes into the back as a spotty youth carried small items down the path. I stopped.

"Er – good morning – um – I know this sounds odd but have you found anything strange in there?" The rough looking man stopped and stared at me, pushing back his cap.

"Strange? We find something strange in every house we clear. People are strange – you wouldn't believe some of the things we've come across. How strange do you mean exactly?"

"Well – er – a coffin?"

"Coffins – let me see – do you mean empty coffins or full coffins?"

"Well – a coffin with a body?"

"No, I can't say as I've noticed any bodies today. Here Shane," he called to his mate, "you seen any bodies in there?"

"Nah – there's a stuffed fox in a glass case. Oh! And a dead mouse under the kitchen sink – will that do?" They both burst out laughing.

"Tell you what, if we find a body we'll let you know," the older man snorted and turned back to his van.

I slunk off feeling very silly. Mrs. Pickles' curtains were twitching and I knew I could safely leave the monitoring of the contents of the house to her 'miss nothing' beady gaze. Meanwhile I made a mental note never to listen to the ramblings of the Mrs Pickles of this world again.

* * *

Gertrude Warhurst was to be an unforgettable patient and one who was to change my life. Following a stroke she had become bed bound in the local geriatric hospital and after three months on ward 14, Gertrude decided she was going home. She lived alone in an invalid unfriendly Victorian terraced house, with many steps, an inadequate heating system, and various other inconveniences.

She was severely disabled and unable to stand and even Dr Sangeet the consultant geriatrician, whose whole life was dedicated to throwing out as many patients as possible, as soon as possible, didn't think Gertrude could be cared for at home alone.

An assessment visit was carried out whereby Gertrude was taken home by ambulance accompanied by an occupational therapist and the geriatric liaison officer to see how well she could cope. She failed miserably but no matter, Gertrude had decided she would go home and she signed the discharge book. However, since she could hardly set off under her own steam, she still needed the consent of the geriatric consultant, and a relative to take responsibility.

Her only relative was Harold, her brother, an odious, argumentative retired civil servant who lived with his equally unpleasant wife about a mile from Gertrude's home. They had visited Gertrude almost daily during her time on ward 14 and had been vociferous in complaining about her care to the ward sisters, matron, the consultant and anyone within earshot. Now Harold's anger was re-directed to complaining about the very idea that she could come home, until he over played his hand and threatened the consultant with the front page of the local paper. Dr Sangeet immediately said he would agree to let Gertrude go home 'on a trial basis.'

As far as Harold's consent was concerned, Gertrude had a trump card up her sleeve and now she played it. As Harold was the sole executor and beneficiary of her will, she told him her will could easily be changed in favour of the cats' home. Harold went pale and hurried home to start making arrangements. The hospital contacted the Community services – home helps, district nurses, meals on wheels and her G.P's. The hospital was ridding itself of two thorns in its sides, and the thorns were about to stick into me.

My first visit was a few hours after Gertrude arrived home. I walked up the fifteen stone steps carrying arms full of incontinence sheets and pads and other nursing aids. Gertrude was sitting in a high chair next to a hospital bed, a commode, and a hoist provided for lifting and handling. I was to visit twice a day. Harold would also visit, and the evening nurses would put her to bed. Before I could tell her my name, she greeted me with –

"I'm glad you're here – I want to go to bed – and I'm not going in that thing." She pointed at the hoist.

Tony, the geriatric liaison officer had warned me she was difficult to handle and without a hoist two nurses were needed. It wasn't so much that Gertrude was fat, she was tall and heavy boned. Even as an old lady she was over six feet tall. This made her difficult to lift and move.

I pointed out to Gertrude that I would find it difficult to get her into bed by myself and reminded her that she had promised the hospital she would use the hoist.

"Never mind what I said in there, I'm at home now and I'm not being bossed around by nurses in my own home!" she snapped.

I undressed her in the chair then struggled to get her from chair to bed, succeeding more by good luck than good management. Back in my office I telephoned the occupational health nurse at the hospital and asked her to meet me at Gertrude's for her opinion as to whether one nurse should be trying to cope on her own and to see if she could persuade her to use the hoist. She was just about to go on holiday for two weeks, but an appointment was made for when she was back.

Meanwhile, we struggled on with me seeking help from colleagues when possible. This was usually given reluctantly or even resentfully and as ever there was no understanding or help to be had from nurse management. There was an unspoken attitude that you were incompetent if you couldn't manage a patient on your own; all well and good when the patient would use a hoist. My shoulders and back began to ache and for the first time I dreaded going to work.

Harold soon started being as difficult as his sister. Large notices began to appear all over the house. Gertrude had a plastic bag attached to her leg into which her urinary catheter drained and one morning it burst as I was changing it. Holding it together as best I could, I made an Olympic dash for the sink in the kitchen, and after disposing of the torn bag I gave the sink a good scrub round with bleach.

"DO NOT PUT URINE DOWN THIS SINK" said the large notice in thick black felt tip, the next day. Although there was no love lost between Harold and Gertrude, she obviously told him tales about us.

To empty Gertrude's commode we had to trail up a long flight of narrow, steep steps to an old fashioned lavatory which had a high water tank and a long chain pull to flush it. It was obviously in need of a plumber, as when flushed, the bowl filled almost to overflowing and the water seeped slowly away accompanied by strange noises and convulsions of large air bubbles.

Unfortunately, Gertrude ate like a horse, anything she could get her hands on. In between her three main meals of the day she consumed biscuits, chocolates and fruit. Consequently, the contents of her commode resembled what a healthy hippopotamus might pass, and the ancient ailing toilet, after struggling manfully for a few weeks, finally gave up the ghost.

I left a note for Harold, who was due with lunch, suggesting that a plumber was needed A.S.A.P., and left the commode pot next to the toilet. At the afternoon visit I read his reply to the effect that the toilet had been alright before nurses had been visiting and he would leave it to me to empty the commode and pull the chain 'properly'.

'DO NOT LEAVE UNEMPTIED EXCRETA NEXT TO THIS TOILET' said the notice as I went to try to comply with his instructions. Thinking 'alright Harold, have it your way', I emptied the hippopotamus sized poo into the bowl and pulled the chain. It was still sitting there stubbornly at the third attempt to flush it away.

After a further exchange of *billets-doux,* he must have got a plumber, as the toilet flushed the following day, but the big notice remained in situ.

Things improved slightly when, after two evening visit staff went off sick with back injuries, Gertrude was informed by a letter from management that she would in future be moved by the hoist. She finally accepted this, no doubt frightened by the thought that we might send her back to hospital, a fear I did nothing to discourage whilst knowing there was virtually no way they would have her back, and we jogged along until the day of my appointment with the occupational health sister dawned. She was an extremely pleasant, practical woman who was married to one of the hospital consultants.

Gertrude accepted her as just another nurse going round with me, and after getting her all done and dusted we sat in Sister Dacre's car for a chat.

"I'm glad some-one has seen sense and made her accept the hoist," she said, "but she still is very hard work for any nurse on her own. At present we can't do anything to help district nurses in these situations but the day is coming when the accent will swing from pandering to the patient to protecting the nurses. Legislation is being brought in under a Health and Safety Executive and nurse managers will have a duty of care to protect their staff. Any nurse who is injured in the workplace will be able to sue their Health Authority. In the future nurses on the district will go round in twos a lot of the time. In the meantime we just have to carry on."

I was grateful for her visit but wondered if I would live to see these miraculous changes. It sounded unbelievable that anyone would be on our side.

I rarely actually bumped into Harold but when I did he was full of complaints about what we were or were not doing. He complained to me about the evening staff and to the evening staff about the day staff. Meanwhile, the notices grew ever more ubiquitous.

'DO NOT PINCH THE MATCHES FROM THIS COOKER. HOW DO YOU EXPECT TO LIGHT IT?'

Underneath some wag had written "I wouldn't dare try – it must be a hundred years old!"

'WIPE YOUR FEET ON THE MAT PROVIDED.'

Although in many ways a total pain, Harold's notices were becoming quite hilarious and none of us took them seriously.

'SOMEONE HAS STOLEN A TOILET ROLL!' – and so it went on until one day I looked at my difficult patient surrounded by Harold's notices and thought, 'well Gertrude, someone is going to have to look after you for years, but it's not going to be me.'

It was the dawning of an idea that maybe I should change my life and it was an exciting idea.

In a few months time I would reach my twenty-one years nursing as a Queen's District Nursing Sister. I was the only one on the area who had been trained under the Queen's system. District nurse training had changed radically over the years and every local authority now trained their own nurses, which made me feel like a dinosaur. Many of the younger girls had never heard of Queen's training. One asked if it was Queen Alexandra's nurses, thinking of the armed forces. "Victoria actually," I mumbled, feeling older than ever.

After twenty one years of service, Queen's nurses were given an enamel badge, presented by a member of the Royal family at a ceremony held once a year in London. In nineteen seventy seven, the Queen's silver jubilee year, her Majesty had presented the badges.

The last recipient from our area was Betty Harrison, about five years previously under the West Riding County Council who were proud of their long serving Queen's nurses. Betty and her husband had gone down to London all expenses paid and an article with Betty's photograph had appeared in two local papers.

Now, following the re-organisation of local government, we were Cowslipdale Area Health Authority, with a new po-faced nursing officer who definitely gave me the impression that neither she nor Cowslipdale wanted to know.

Mrs Stead, the health department office manager, was outraged on my behalf.

"Mrs Harrison received congratulations from the Chief Nurse of the West Riding and the Medical Officer of Health and was told to go and enjoy her day in London. Why don't you just go and give me your expenses claim Sister Baines?"

I decided I would, and I asked Shirley, my sister-in-law to accompany me. We met at Halifax station and enjoyed our train ride to Kings Cross. We walked through the city, past St Paul's Cathedral to the Fishmonger's Hall, where the ceremony was to be held, the badges to be presented by Her Royal Highness the Dowager Duchess of Gloucester.

At the top of some marble stairs we entered two large reception rooms, beautifully decorated in red and gold with gilt mirrors and magnificent chandeliers. Three or four elderly officials of the Queen's Institute clutching clipboards were ticking us off and generally bossing everyone about. In our well pressed uniforms we checked out hats were on straight and our gloves were spotless. The relatives and friends accompanying us were sent to sit at one side of the room and we sat on gilt and red velvet chairs at the other side. We all had to be in place about half an hour before Her Royal Highness was due to arrive.

Comparing notes with my neighbour on the left, we found we had both had Miss Healey as our examiner twenty-one years ago.

"My exam was a nightmare," I said

"Oh I bet I can top it," she said, "I'd spent weeks arranging everything but I had to drag my first patient out of the pub, and my last one had decided to commit suicide and was lying in the kitchen with her head in the gas oven."

I thought I could safely say – that topped it.

Soon, we were moving out in rows to receive our badges from the Dowager Duchess. She was beautifully dressed and charming and with a quick handshake, a curtsey and a flash of a camera it was all over. We met up with our friends and relatives at the bar in the next room for drinks and nibbles. Following a late lunch in a sandwich bar, Shirley and I caught the train home.

Back in the office Mrs Stead was eager to hear all about it as she took my receipts to submit to the treasurer. Five days later I was summoned to my new nursing officer's room.

"What is this about Sister Baines?" she waived my expenses claim under my nose.

In short, she was not impressed by my Queen's District Nursing Institute twenty-one years service award. As far as how previous recipients had been treated she didn't give a stuff and it was made clear that I was a very naughty nurse and my expenses would not be paid. This ran off me like water off a duck's back as it was more or less what I had expected. Nurse managers had always behaved in ridiculously autocratic ways and I had never expected this to change in my working life time.

A few months later this new broom decided she would make her mark and sweep clean with a vengeance. She decided she would uproot us all and move us all round. Long standing working relationships with our doctors counted for nothing. The fact that most of us lived on or near our areas counted for nothing either – in fact that was probably the problem. She was lying awake at night worrying that since we were near home we might pop in for a cuppa and put our feet up for ten minutes.

What she had given no consideration to was that Cowslipdale was a very hilly area and when it snowed heavily, as it did every winter, ill patients or those needing vital injections could usually be reached somehow by a nurse who lived on her area. To have to drive miles every day to and fro, all passing each other on the way, seemed madness. Most of my colleagues were upset and up in arms about it, and one or two seemed to be hovering on the edge of a nervous breakdown. However, when it came to doing something about it, standing up to be counted, most of them had an excuse.

"I've only three, four, five years to go before I get my pension – I'm not sticking my neck out," was the one most commonly heard.

Four of us decided to risk all and invoke the grievance procedure and inform our professional body the Royal College of Nursing. Po-face was astounded. She hadn't reckoned on this. We became known as the 'gang of four', as four politicians who had founded the Liberal Democrats were known.

Meetings were called at the Health Department which were attended by we four rebels, senior nursing staff from the Area Health Authority and our Royal College of Nursing representative, a rather wimpish young man with an Oxford accent, called Colin, who carried an impressive leather brief case which we suspected contained little more than marmite sandwiches which his mum had made.

Win, a spirited girl from the Eastham area was more or less our ring leader. She was an excellent district nurse who had given sterling service as a Practical Work Teacher for twenty years. Her patients adored her and she was greatly respected by doctors and nursing colleagues alike. However, on this occasion she had really set the cat among the pigeons by giving an interview to the press.

'*Nurses in revolt over staff movements*', said the headlines in the local evening paper. '*Cowslipdale nurse managers in battle with Union*' said a leader in the Bridgend Echo, whilst the item which most enraged the powers that be was a photograph of a motley bunch of patients waving placards which said '*Don't move our Win! Leave our district nurses alone!*" – the headline being '*Win hopes to win the day.*'

Our respective doctors all wrote to the management saying they were more than satisfied with 'their' nurse and didn't want the upheaval of having to get used to a new nurse as they saw it as unnecessary. My lot loyally wrote of me in glowing terms, which was no doubt done during the morning break, as they had managed to get coffee stains and jam smudges on it.

Finally, not wanting further trouble or publicity, management backed down. We four realised we would be forever in the bad books but as that was the style of management anyway, what was new?

We should have known better as they merely waited a few months for the dust to settle then renewed their plans, this time only moving the four of us and the four who would take our places. Our 'mole' at the Health Department sent us all a copy of a memo to Po-face from the Chief Nurse Manager. Win was to be sent to the roughest area of Cowslipdale. Susie was to be banished to Todmorden and Jill could stay where she was as long as she took Susie's patch as well as her own!

The last sentence said, 'Sister Baines is needed where she is at present, due to sickness, but will be dealt with at a later date.'

I sat in my car with a beef sandwich, which I suddenly felt would choke me, digesting the words 'will be dealt with', and suddenly I knew I would not give them the satisfaction of 'dealing' with me. It was time to review my working life. A few days later I saw a job advertised in the local paper for a Practice Nurse at a three doctor practice a few miles down the valley. Practice nursing was in it's infancy and was a bit of a leap in the dark but I would apply.

I thoroughly enjoyed a friendly interview with two very pleasant young doctors but I had no great hopes of being offered the job as there were several candidates and the one who came out as I went in was very glamorous, dressed stylishly in mufti with high heels and wearing full make up.

The doctors understood the problems we had with nurse management. Their district nurse was frequently 'ambushed' by her nurse manager, who lay in wait up a side street to see what time she headed for home! Their questions were not too onerous and at least they didn't ask if my oven switched itself on!

The following day the practice manager rang to offer me the job. With some glee I informed Po-face, who sounded quite miffed that she had missed out on 'dealing' with me. As I worked my notice I found it a time for reflection. Taking it all into account I'd had a great time 'on the district' and so many people, colleagues, carers and patients would always have a place in my heart.

My last patient of course had to be Gertrude Warhurst. This is the last time I'm going to do this I thought happily, as Gertrude swung in mid air in her hoist, surrounded by Harold's notices.

I was off to pastures new. How exciting life was!